LANGUAGE STRATEGIES FOR CHILDREN

KEYS TO CLASSROOM SUCCESS

Vicki Prouty, M.S., CCC-SLP

Michele Fagan, M.S., CCC-SLP

Super Duper® Publications • Greenville, South Carolina

10 09 10 9 8 7 6

Library of Congress Cataloging-in-Publication Data

Prouty, Vicki
Language strategies for children : keys to classroom success / Vicki Prouty. Michele Fagan.
p. cm.
Includes bibliographical references.
ISBN 1-888222-01-8 (pbk.)
1. Speech therapy for children--Problems, exercises, etc. 2. Language arts--Problems, exercises, etc. 3. Children--Language--Problems, exercises, etc. 4. Language experience approach in education--Problems, exercises. etc. I. Fagan, Michele, II. Title.
LB3454.F34 1997 97-9031
371.91'4--dc21 CIP

Printed in the United States of America

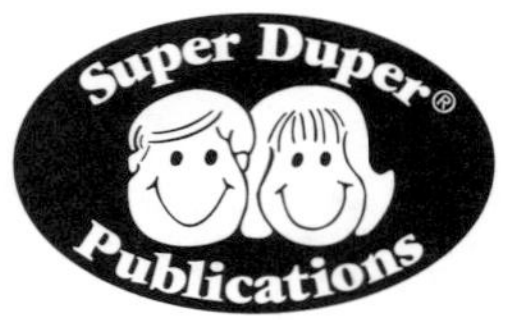

Super Duper® Publications
Post Office Box 24997 • Greenville, South Carolina 29616 USA
www.superduperinc.com
Call 1-800-277-8737 • Fax 1-800-978-7379

To our husbands, who waited patiently
as we spent countless hours in front of a computer screen

CONTENTS

PREFACE

Although we did not know it at the time, the *Language Strategies for Children* project began five years ago when the speech-language pathologists in our school district began experimenting with alternative service delivery models. Because our schools were similar in size, caseload, and location, we opted to pilot a "teaming" approach.

There were several ways that teaming improved the quality and efficiency of our teaching. We shared caseloads and/or schedules which allowed for doubling up the number of students seen during a particular block of time. Scheduling flexibility was wonderful, since one of us could be in the classroom while the other worked in small groups elsewhere. Teaming also allowed for shared planning time. When planning together, we discovered that we had complementary teaching styles and approaches. While one of us might have been thinking about a lesson from a visual standpoint, the other was more sequential. Having once taught a lesson, we would keep notes to improve it, and then by comparing notes, the lessons evolved into well-rounded teaching tools. Finally, this process led to developing a plan for avoiding redundancy while covering the key objectives of our program.

We are so thankful that we took the risk in trying a teaming approach. Ideas continue to blossom and we truly do enjoy the opportunity to collaborate with each other.

Special thanks are extended to Dr. Alan Bird, of Texas Women's University, who got us started with the teaming idea. Thanks also to the supportive personnel at Wells and Saigling Elementary Schools of Plano, for their input and collaboration with us in their classrooms, and to the students who continue to help us grow and learn each day. We also thank our reviewers—Sue Schultz, Linda Roth, Vicki Lord Larson, Beth Hibbard, and Nancy Lund—whose suggestions have helped to improve this book.

INTRODUCTION

OVERVIEW

Since 1990, the inclusion movement has prompted a shift in focus for providing special services to children with exceptional needs. In considering the "least restrictive environment" provision of the Individuals with Disabilities Education Act (IDEA), educators are part of a movement to provide services within the classroom setting when appropriate. Naremore (1995) terms this service delivery as *classroom-based intervention.* The speech-language pathologist or learning disabilities specialist provides services in the classroom, sometimes teaching alongside the classroom teacher and sometimes building around or supplementing the lessons being taught in the classroom (Naremore, 1995). It is as important as ever to ensure students are successful in the classroom setting. Students need strategies for success. The strategies presented in *Language Strategies for Children: Keys to Classroom Success* are appropriate for classroom-based intervention.

Language Strategies for Children is a multifaceted tool for developing the communication skills of students in grades two through five. The lessons integrate whole language philosophy, classroom curriculum concepts, literature-based intervention techniques, and strategies for self-prompting. This resource capitalizes on students' visual strengths by providing creative, visual reminders of strategies. Memorable strategy names help students internalize strategy use. Use of the strategies in other settings is encouraged through homework assignments, vacation calendar activities, and the creation of booklets.

Language Strategies for Children embeds Hunter's (1982) lesson cycle format and the principles of brain-based research discussed by Caine and Caine (1991) and Kavalic and Olsen (1993). It provides activities that will appeal to students with different learning styles so that each child has an opportunity for success in learning about communication. As a way to reach students with learning problems, Rief (1993) proposes the use of multisensory methods to promote high interest, relevancy, and motivation. In addition, these methods stress active participation and interaction among peers. Multisensory methods are applied throughout the *Language Strategies for Children* lessons.

Communication goals focus on three primary categories: (1) language comprehension, (2) oral expression, and (3) story grammar knowledge, which to enhance remembrance will be called simply "story knowledge" in the lessons. An organizational chart (see page 15) cross-references individual lessons to lesson objectives. Engaging literature is integral to teaching the goals and objectives. Creative links to curriculum through literature (e.g., the book *Barn Dance!* [Martin and Archambault, 1986] lends itself to a discussion of the curriculum concepts *urban* and *rural*) make *Language Strategies for Children* an ideal tool for schools implementing an inclusion model. Activities are interactive and include reading, writing, role-playing, and art. Adapting lessons for small groups versus classroom settings and suggestions for varying lessons are included.

Program Goals

Four major goals are emphasized in *Language Strategies for Children*:

1. To provide students with multisensory strategies that
   - promote self-learning and self-prompting;
   - decrease the need for direct assistance from an adult; and
   - help students experience success in the least restrictive classroom environment.
2. To help students recognize responsibility for their learning by
   - teaching goal setting as a means of increased ownership and self-improvement;
   - providing a framework for self-evaluation; and
   - demonstrating the application of goals in classroom and home settings.
3. To encourage parent participation by
   - increasing awareness of their child's program and goals; and
   - providing quick, easy, home-related communication activities.
4. To monitor progress by
   - utilizing authentic assessment to track progress over time (e.g., collecting work in a portfolio); and
   - measuring independent use of strategies for mastery of communication goals.

Intended Users

Language Strategies for Children can be used in small group settings and in large groups or in classrooms. Educators who strive for students to become independent learners and generalizers of skills in the classroom, at home, and eventually in work environments will find this resource useful. Strategies for learning are appropriate for all students, though the primary focus of this resource is students with learning difficulties. The lessons are appropriate for students in grades two through five, or those who are functioning at that level developmentally. Although most activities are written for group participation, the strategy lessons could be adapted for remediation of students with language disorders or learning disabilities on an individual basis.

BACKGROUND

Language Strategies for Children is based on several educational models, principles, and philosophies that address the needs of the learner as a whole. These premises are embedded within the lessons.`

Repeated Exposure

Caine and Caine (1991), Kavalic and Olsen (1993), and Hunter (1982) describe natural brain functioning and the implications for the teaching process. The teaching principles suggested by these researchers stress the uniqueness and total emotional, physiological, and psychological involvement of the brain in the learning process, particularly the need to pair familiarity with novelty and challenge and the need for repeated exposure. The brain's search for meaning through "patterning" (i.e., patterns connect new knowledge to prior experience) is an important learning component (Caine and Caine, 1991; Kavalic and Olsen, 1993).

Multisensory Methods

Rief (1993) reports that the majority of students are visual and tactile/kinesthetic learners. She cautions, "Only 15 percent tend to be strong auditory learners. If your teaching style emphasizes lecturing, with you doing all the talking, there is a high percentage of students you're not reaching... We need to present lessons with a combination of methods" (p. 53). The lessons in *Language Strategies for Children* provide activities that appeal to students with different learning styles so that each student has an opportunity and an avenue for success in language learning. Sounds, words, or rhymes are highlighted to engage the auditory learner. Students have the opportunity to practice communicating in meaningful contexts and interactions. Visual learners have the benefit of a visual aid or graphic representation of the strategy. Clapping, tracing, and gesturing are utilized for the tactile/kinesthetic learner. Children have opportunities for pragmatic (social skill) practice in both large and small group activities. Other subject areas can be integrated into the lessons to draw on potential student strengths (e.g., math, science, music). For example, while giving or receiving directions in the *barrier map* activity, the numbers of correct responses can be tallied or calculated into percentages by particular students. In this way, a student who may not be an effective communicator, but excels in math, may have a chance to be successful.

Strategy-Based Intervention

Language Strategies for Children presents strategies for learning. The strategies require students to self-evaluate and self-monitor their communication skills. For students who experience communication breakdowns in social situations (e.g., when talking with friends), or at school (e.g., when listening to the teacher or working on class projects within a group), or who find vocabulary or concepts in classroom curricula challenging, strategies provide a plan for repairing the interactions when breakdown occurs. Cognitive (e.g., analyzing) and metacognitive (e.g., planning and organizing) strategies are important to effective language learning (Oxford, 1994). Strategies should fit learning styles and language tasks (i.e., they should be multisensory and meet the needs of visual symbolizers as well as auditory symbolizers [McInroy, 1996]). There should be plenty of opportunity for practicing strategies during the language lesson. The teaching of strategies should include explanations, handouts, activities, and home practice materials (Oxford, 1994).

Language Strategies for Children is a strategy-based program. For example, if a student is learning to write descriptively, a tactile strategy for self-prompting descriptive words is taught. In the *It Makes Sense* lesson, the strategy is to have the students place their thumb on their ear, their pointer finger on their eye, their middle finger on their nose, their ring finger on their mouth, and their little finger on one's chin to represent touch, thus using all of the senses tactilely to create a description. Each strategy has an accompanying visual graphic, an activity for learning it, an opportunity for demonstrating use of the strategy, and homework activities for family involvement.

Whole Language Philosophy

Whole language has been described as a partnership between intent and learning, focusing on meaning and relevancy as the catalyst for learning (Wagner, 1989). Whole language capitalizes on the social aspects of communication in which the language learner strives to bridge experiences and understanding (Genishi, 1988). While the whole language philosophy is not applied in its purest form in *Language Strategies for Children,* language learning is addressed in context, as it occurs, in "language-loaded" situations. Lessons integrate listening, speaking, reading, and writing at a level appropriate to the student.

Curriculum-Based Intervention

Intervention that integrates curriculum vocabulary and concepts with communication goals is termed *curriculum-based intervention* (A. Bird, personal communication, September 1, 1992). This approach to intervention creates a relevant context for language learning. *Language Strategies for Children* is curriculum-based. For example, maps are used to practice using clear, specific language when giving directions to a partner. The message sender places a number of items on his or her map and gives directions for placement to a partner whose view is blocked by a barrier. Concepts and vocabulary include: *north, south, east, west, above, below, mountain, valley, hill, river, lake, near, far, right,* and *left*. This activity clearly emphasizes use of specific language and requesting clarification when further information is needed while incorporating relevant subject matter. It is important to keep in mind that curriculum-based and classroom-based intervention emphasizes communication goals, not the curriculum content, but uses curricular concepts as the stimuli for improving communication. Educators should adapt activities by embedding their district's curriculum goals and objectives into the lessons.

Literature-Based Intervention

Language Strategies for Children embeds literature of high interest, which is an engaging, entertaining format for learning communication. For example, *Roxaboxen* (1991) by Barbara Cooney lends itself to teaching categorization. It tells the story of children who pretend that an abandoned lot on a hillside is a community. The children use the rubble, rocks, desert glass, and plants to create an outline in the desert sand of houses, streets, shops, and businesses. Students expand on the ideas learned from the story to categorize the many parts of a community, such as occupations, transportation, goods and services, etc. *Language Strategies for Children* lessons incorporate literature that can be linked to the classroom curriculum. The literature used in *Language Strategies for Children* is listed in the bibliography.

Portfolio Assessment

A longitudinal approach to assessment combines alternative views of the students' performance for a more complete view of achievement (Herman, Aschbacher, and Winters, 1992). A *portfolio* is a systematic way to assess student work longitudinally. The student work selected provides information about the student's level of development and growth over time (Grace, 1992). A variety of information can be made available in portfolios, such as what the child has learned and how the child goes about learning. Portfolios can provide information about how the child processed, analyzed, and synthesized what was learned. Portfolios provide benchmarks for quality that the student can review to see improvement over time. Well-planned portfolios include work in progress and "showpiece" samples (Herman, Aschbacher, and Winters, 1992). Portfolios provide a framework for authentic assessment where observations of work performance, as well as products collected from spontaneous and planned samples, can be evaluated. Children are motivated toward quality as soon as they discover that their work will be "shown" or highlighted as part of their portfolio.

Grace (1992) describes two options for collecting the samples: (1) collect samples the students take home at the end of the year, and (2) collect samples that stay at school for a "school career" portfolio. This second type of portfolio may be shared with parents at conference time or at an annual review meeting. This is the model that *Language Strategies for Children* suggests. Work samples and teacher observations are documented throughout the year to show growth and mastery of strategy knowledge. This information can be kept in students' portfolios. Students' goal sheets can also be collected and kept in their portfolios.

PROGRAM COMPONENTS

Lessons

Hunter's (1982) lesson cycle format further reinforces the principles of brain-based research by providing repeated exposure to a concept within a lesson. Hunter describes the lesson components she feels maximize learning on the part of the student. The lesson components include the following:

1. *Objectives*—describe the change in student behavior that is desired;
2. *Anticipatory Set*—sets the stage for learning by sparking student interest and curiosity about the lesson;
3. *Modeling*—presents examples of behaviors the educator wants the students to perform independently;
4. *Guided Practice*—checks the students' level of understanding of the concept before moving on; and,
5. *Independent Practice*—provides tasks to be completed until students show mastery of the lesson concepts or skills.

The lesson format used in *Language Strategies for Children: Keys to Classroom Success* is an adaptation of Hunter's (1982) model. In addition to *Goal, Background Information,* and *Materials,* every lesson includes the following components:

1. *Objectives*—The objectives clearly state the change expected in students' behavior within each lesson, although measurable elements should be added based on each individual's needs.
2. *Introduction*—The introduction parallels the anticipatory set of Hunter's (1982) model. It has two elements, *tie-in to prior learning* and *focus/relevancy*. The *tie-in to prior learning* is a review of the previous lesson (if appropriate). It sets the stage for connecting prior experience with new knowledge. The *focus/relevancy* section establishes an anticipatory set. Therefore, more meaningful or vivid entry into a topic results. Focusing techniques include a proposal of a provocative question or a statement of the objective. The purpose of this component is to have students clear their minds of irrelevant ideas and be ready to learn, especially since they know what it is they are to focus on and what they are expected to learn.

3. *Lesson Activities*—The lesson activity presents the basic information necessary to meet the objectives. Modeling the strategy or process is essential to ensuring understanding. Hunter (1982) stresses the use of key words and simple diagrams in a lesson and these techniques are what comprise the language strategies presented. Each lesson activity includes checking for understanding, including signaled answers, choral responses, or a sampling of individual responses (either oral or written).

4. *Closure*—The closure activity includes a discussion of the lesson relevance and value. "Teaching for transfer," as Hunter (1982) calls it, involves making the information meaningful by connecting past and future knowledge to present learning. The educator identifies critical parts of the present learning and ties it to the child's life, using techniques such as mnemonics or memory helpers. "Teaching for meaning" (i.e., introducing short meaningful "chunks" of information for students to practice), as Hunter terms it, is included through guided and independent practice.

Lessons also apply the principle of "distributed practice" in that strategies previously taught are revisited periodically as they apply to a current lesson to improve retention of the strategy. For example, the lesson on analogies applies the strategies for synonyms and antonyms, comparing and contrasting, classification, listening actively, and drawing conclusions.

Strategy Graphic

Each strategy has a graphic visual aid. The graphic should be duplicated and enlarged to create a poster. The poster can be colored and laminated for durability. It should be posted on a classroom wall or bulletin board and referred to while students are learning the strategy or when the strategy is reviewed.

The graphic can also be used to create transparencies for overhead projectors. For example, in the *Compare Contrastadon* lesson, the educator could use the transparency to write on while comparing and contrasting two objects or concepts. The transparencies could also be used to generalize strategy use to curriculum concepts throughout the day.

Goal Setting

Language Strategies for Children stresses responsibility and ownership of communication goals. For each of the three units, students write self-directed goals with the help of the educator and form their own plans for improvement. Students think about why the goals are relevant at school, at home, and in other situations and write their thoughts on their goal sheets. Within each unit, after several strategies have been taught, students complete a new goal sheet. Students decide whether or not they have achieved the previous goal or how they could revise their plan to ensure better progress; they record their progress and think about the new goal.

The goal sheets are taken home so students can share their goals with family members. While students will develop skills at school, some of the practice has to occur at home so students achieve their goals. Goal sheets serve as documentation of progress and help communicate progress to family members. Goal sheets should be signed by family members and returned. (A reward could be earned for returning the signed goal sheets.)

Goal setting is an extremely successful and motivational teaching strategy. Students feel informed about their program and progress and are therefore more enthusiastic and motivated. This is demonstrated by the change in students' attitudes and performance.

Strategy Pages

A two-page strategy guide is provided for each strategy in this resource. These pages are compiled to form a *Strategy Guide Booklet*. Each time a new strategy is learned, the strategy guide pages are completed and added to the booklet. At the end of the school year, students have a collection of information regarding skills and strategies learned. Each strategy guide includes the strategy graphic and a summary of the strategy. The second page of each strategy guide asks the students to write about how the strategy helped or could help in real-life situations. The settings students consider are home, school, and community.

Homework Activities

A homework activity is also provided for each strategy so that students can share the targeted skill and strategy with their families. The homework activity includes the strategy graphic and the skill being learned. The homework activities ask students to share the strategy with their family members and then apply the strategy to several tasks at home. If students complete this activity, family members are asked to sign the sheet and return it to school. Establishing a reward system for completing the activity and returning signed sheets helps to ensure this important step is done.

The homework activities encourage parent/child involvement and give family members examples of how home practice can support communication skills in a quick, easy, and useful way. Students learn that their parents value good communication skills.

Portfolios

For this resource, goal sheets, strategy guide pages, returned homework activity pages, and anecdotal information regarding progress or concerns comprise the students' portfolios. The educator should collect these items, as well as relevant classroom work, to keep in the portfolios. Anecdotal notes from a variety of teachers are a valuable source of documentation of progress as the child moves from grade to grade. The notes could give specific examples of when students apply strategies (e.g., a teacher may document that on 1/12, Jimmy did not request help with his math assignment, got frustrated, and did not complete it on 2/23, Jimmy asked for clarification about his math assignment and then went on to complete it). These anecdotes may also be obtained by briefly interviewing teachers regarding their observations of a student's growth over time.

Educator-created checklists to itemize desired communication skills or strategy use may also be used to assess progress informally. A child's current performance may be compared to his or her previous performances (work samples, pre- and posttesting, and anecdotal information) to show change over time. Portfolio collections should be shared with family members and students at annual meetings or parent-teacher conferences.

Vacation Calendar

Language Strategies for Children includes a *Vacation Calendar*. The calendar includes two months worth of activities that can be done in five minutes or less on a daily basis at home. If using the calendar in a "traditional," nine-month school year, the activities could be completed during the summer months. If using the calendar in a year-round school district, the calendar is easily adapted to accommodate such a schedule.

The months and dates are purposely not included on the calendar to allow flexibility, but should be added before duplicating for students. Educators should recommend to students, or to family members at an annual review meeting or conference, that the calendar be hung on the refrigerator (or some other prominent spot) and worked on at a specific time each day (e.g., breakfast or bedtime). Parents or caregivers should initial each daily activity when it is completed. A reward for completed and signed calendars may be offered at the beginning of the return to school.

PROCEDURES FOR USE

Language Strategies for Children is written as the starting point for educators who will develop lessons into their own style of teaching. It provides a framework that a beginning teacher can follow or one that an experienced teacher can incorporate into a previously existing program. The lessons will spur new ideas.

Units and Goals

Language Strategies for Children is divided into three main units. The units generally focus on three areas: (1) language comprehension, (2) oral expression, and (3) story grammar knowledge.

1. *Language Comprehension*—addresses the listening process by:
    - making the student aware of the difference between hearing and listening (i.e., one can hear sounds in the environment, but until the brain is engaged, no meaning is attached to the sound source)
    - discussing what can interfere (both intrinsically and extrinsically) with the listening process
    - discussing what to do in distracting situations
    - building active listening skills during lessons (The students are frequently given a listening job [i.e., specific information or words to listen for] to keep them involved and focused.)
    - stressing evaluative thinking (The lessons create opportunities for students to recognize the need for clarification as well as how to ask for clarification appropriately.)
    - applying evaluative listening and thinking skills to differentiate fact from opinion in a variety of contexts.
2. *Oral Expression*—addresses the speaking process by:
    - stressing the use of the five senses to describe objects, pictures, and events
    - discussing the use of descriptive language in creating a more vivid message for the listener (or reader, if written)
    - discussing the need to make scientific observations and to verbally share discoveries with other observers on a team
    - emphasizing the use of precise and specific language terms in communication (e.g., antonyms and synonyms, spatial relationships)
    - emphasizing the use of communication skills in problem solving and higher level thinking (e.g., identifying analogous patterns, categorizing, recognizing part-whole relationships)
    - teaching the parts of speech (e.g., noun, verb, adjective) for use in manipulating language meaning (e.g., in using multiple meanings of words, figurative language, creative and original expression, and in giving clear, precise definitions).

3. *Story Grammar Knowledge*—addresses narrative language skills by:

   - providing a guideline of story grammar elements
   - stressing the use of a story grammar framework for relaying a personal experience or generating or retelling a fictional story
   - applying story grammar strategies to oral and written language
   - emphasizing the need to tell the important points rather than retelling an entire story when summarizing or giving the main idea
   - applying evaluative listening/thinking skills to link information and recognize the parts of a cause/effect relationship.

Communication objectives are organized within these three units. Lessons clearly emphasize one of the three areas of communication described above, however in keeping with the philosophy of whole language, all areas of communication are integrated within lessons (i.e., a lesson with a listening goal may also contain objectives with a speaking focus).

The Cross-Reference Chart (see page 15) lists the objectives covered in each lesson. While several objectives are targeted specifically, a number of objectives are indirectly developed as well. In this way, the lessons build upon one another, with previous objectives reviewed in subsequent lessons. This repetition also accommodates the needs of students who enter the program at different times and may have missed earlier lessons.

Presenting the Lesson

The lessons are presented for use in a classroom setting; however, they are easily adapted for smaller groups by allowing more individual responses and participation. Using the lessons within a small group setting allows the educator to spend whatever time is necessary to ensure that all students have an understanding of the targeted objectives. A small group setting also provides more opportunities for independent practice.

Lessons are taught to second through fifth graders. Content should be expanded and modified within each lesson to fit the particular levels of the students (e.g., when teaching analogies, some students may easily identify the patterns or relationships and can move on to completing an analogy, and then generating their own analogies to fit a particular pattern). The use of higher level questioning can be used to extend any lesson. Bloom's (1956) taxonomy lists a hierarchy of questioning difficulty, beginning at the knowledge level, where only content questions are asked (e.g., "What was the name of the main character?"

"Who was at the party?"). Questions requiring more thought to respond, and questions that require students to manipulate information, arrive at conclusions, or draw inferences (e.g., "Why did John decide to leave?" "Do you agree or disagree with his decision?" "What would his other alternatives be?") should be asked to expand the lesson for older youth.

Most lessons can be taught within a 30-minute class period. However, lessons can be extended over several class periods to ensure understanding or to give students more opportunities to practice a new strategy. Lessons with more than one activity may require more than one session to complete.

Hints are included in many of the lessons to provide helpful information or suggestions for adapting the lessons in different ways. The hints also facilitate the flow of the lesson and are provided to help prevent potential problems.

Suggestions for using literature are included and are referred to as *highlighting literary components.* They are included whenever a piece of literature, listed in the *Materials* section, is used within the lesson. When using any type of literature, the author, illustrator, book cover, and any relevant vocabulary should be discussed. Note particular components of the book while reading the story rather than discussing them out of context before reading the story (e.g., a figurative language expression, multiple meaning words). Suggestions are provided for before reading, during reading, and/or after story reading. If substituting another story, adapt the suggestions for the selected book.

Before beginning any lesson, materials should be gathered. This includes creating the strategy poster, which provides a visual cue for students to remember each targeted strategy. It is an integral part of the lesson and can be referred to in subsequent lessons. The educator should duplicate and enlarge the poster, color it if desired, mount it onto colorful construction paper or poster board, and laminate it for durability. Certain lessons will require the students or educator to write on the poster itself. If laminating is not an option, an overhead transparency of the strategy would allow words to be written and erased easily. Certain parts of the lesson require writing information where all students can see it. In the materials section of each lesson, chalkboard and chalk are listed as the medium for writing the information but a dry erase board or an overhead projector and markers work just as well.

Certain parts of the lessons have been scripted to give the educator an example of presenting the idea. The scripts are examples only and should be reworded to fit the educator's teaching style and the students' learning needs. The scripts, for example, in the *focus/relevancy* section of the lesson are intended to lure the students into the lesson so that they are curious, excited, ready to problem solve, and immediately engaged in the lesson. The educator may opt for a more direct focus by simply stating the purpose of the lesson for the students.

A strategy guide is provided for each strategy presented. The authors have had success with teaching two strategies and then using the corresponding strategy guide lessons as a review. The *Strategy Guide Booklet* is created by adding pages each time a strategy is reviewed, so that at the end of the school term, students have a collection of information regarding the strategies and skills learned. The first page of each strategy guide summarizes the strategy and the skill, and has students demonstrate their understanding of the strategy. The second page of each strategy guide asks students to write about how the strategy helped or could help in real-life situations.

Homework activity sheets are also provided so that the students can share the targeted strategies and skills with their families. The activities generally ask the students to summarize the strategy and apply it to a home or community situation (e.g., help mom classify items on the grocery list). This encourages parent/child involvement and gives family members examples of how home practice can support communication skills in a quick, easy way.

Additional Techniques

The following techniques, occasionally mentioned within the lessons, are methods the authors have found useful when teaching in an inclusion model classroom:

1. *Golf Clap*—The golf clap involves tapping the first two fingers on the palm of the opposite hand. This noiseless clap can be used by an entire class to clap out the syllables in a multisyllabic word when it's difficult to pronounce. It can also be used to show understanding of a concept, as when one student has been called on to give an answer, other students can indicate that they were thinking of the same answer by using their golf clap. The educator can keep more students engaged by acknowledging those students signaling identical responses with their golf clap (e.g., "I see that John and Sara were thinking the same answer as Tom"). The educator may extend responses by asking for different answers or ideas.

2. *Brainstorming*—Brainstorming involves having students generate as many ideas as possible. Ideas are not judged as appropriate or inappropriate when brainstorming because implausible responses can generate alternatives.

3. *Choral Response*—These responses are done in unison as a large group.

4. *Whisper Voices*—The whisper voice is used when the entire classroom is responding in unison in a choral response. The whisper voice minimizes disruption or disturbance of nearby classrooms.

5. *Six-Inch Voices*—Using six-inch voices is a way to describe the volume students should use when working in small groups or pairs. Six-inch voices are voices that can only be heard six inches away. This technique helps to keep the volume level in the classroom manageable.

6. *Learning Groups*—For maximum student participation, many activities suggest students work in small groups. If the educator is versed in the principles of cooperative learning (Johnson, Johnson, and Johnson Holubec, 1990), these principles can be applied. When working in small groups, one student should act as recorder and another as reporter. The recorder records the group's ideas and the reporter shares the ideas with the large group. These roles can be assigned by the group or to save time, the educator can suggest the roles by saying something like, "Today the students wearing the most blue will be the recorders and the students wearing the most brown will be the reporters." This type of strategy gives all group members the opportunity to participate in each role.

CROSS-REFERENCE CHART

The chart on page 15 provides a cross-reference of lessons or strategies and communication goals or objectives. The chart lists the lessons/strategies and goals/objectives targeted within the lessons. (Objectives are stated more specifically within the lessons.) The chart also lists objectives that are indirectly targeted within the lessons. Use this cross-reference to develop goals and objectives for students' individualized educational programs (IEPs) if desired. To use objectives for IEPs, measurable components should be added to the objectives.

Cross-Reference Chart

GOALS/OBJECTIVES \ LESSONS/STRATEGIES	UNIT 1	Give Me Five	CARE	Hit the Bull's-Eye	Detect the Clues	UNIT 2	Creature Creator	It Makes Sense	Lasso the Word Herd	Compare Contrastadon	Weigh the Meaning	Discover the Pattern	Focus for Clarity	Chameleon Words	UNIT 3	Story Recipe	Tell the Biggest Eggs	Follow the Detail Trail
Listening Actively		x	x	x	x		•		•	•	•	•	•	•		•	•	•
Drawing Conclusions		•	•	•	x		•	•	•	•		x		•		•	•	•
Asking Questions (Requesting Clarification)			x	x			x							•				
Making Associations (Comparing and Contrasting)		•	•		x			•	x	x	x	x	•	•		•		
Giving Attributes			•	x			x	x		x	•		x	•				
Categorizing									x	x	•	•	x	•				
Giving Synonyms		•						•	•		x	x	x			•		
Giving Antonyms										x	x	x						
Telling Multiple Meanings		•							•					x		•	•	•
Solving Analogies												x						
Sequencing Events									•							x	x	
Recognizing/Telling Cause and Effect										•						•	•	x
Recognizing and Applying Story Construction																x	x	x
Distinguishing Fact from Opinion					x				•				•					
Telling Main Idea									•							•	x	x
Identifying or Giving Parts of Speech													x	x				
Explaining/Using Figurative Language		•	•				•						•	x		•	•	•
Making Pragmatic Decisions (Using Social Language)		•	•	x			•			•						•		
Demonstrating Knowledge Orally		•	x	x	x		x	x	x	x	x	x	x	x		x	x	x
Demonstrating Knowledge in Written Language					x		x	x	x	x	x	•	x	x		x	x	

x = Targeted objective • = Additional skill that is "touched on" within the lesson

UNIT ONE

GOAL SETTING ACTIVITY ONE

GOAL

To encourage self-improvement through goal setting

BACKGROUND INFORMATION

The main focus of the goal-setting lessons is to help students learn the steps for goal setting (i.e., identifying a need, formulating a goal, practicing the steps to reach the goal, revising a goal as needed, and evaluating progress toward meeting a goal). Rather than expecting students to set goals independently, the goal-setting process is modeled. The communication goal could be teacher directed, but the reflection on how the goal might be useful will be individual for each student, since each student's use of the skills will be different. A few example goals for this unit are:

1. Identify strategies needed for better listening; and
2. Practice strategies for better listening.

OBJECTIVES

1. Understand the vocabulary terms: *goal, skills, achieve.*
2. Become aware of the importance of practicing specific skills in a variety of settings.
3. Write a goal related to listening and identify the importance of listening at home, at school, and in the community.

MATERIALS

1. *My Goals #1* (See page 21; duplicate one per student.)
2. Chalkboard and chalk
3. Pencils

INTRODUCTION

Tie-in to Prior Learning

Discuss with students the idea that when we learn to do something new, it can be hard at first but gets easier with practice. Elicit tasks that require a number of steps to practice, such as blowing a bubble, dribbling a soccer ball, or playing a musical instrument. Relate these tasks to setting, practicing, and achieving a goal that requires learning several skills (e.g., throwing/catching/hitting the ball, and running the bases, etc. to become a good softball player).

Focus/Relevancy

1. Ask who in the class can tell the steps to blowing a bubble with bubble gum. Allow time for response and discuss briefly.

2. Stress that learning is easier when goals are set and steps for achieving them are planned. Each step requires a "strategy" for practicing. Setting goals and learning strategies to reach the goal can help students achieve and accomplish many different skills, both in school and at home.

LESSON ACTIVITIES

1. Give each student a copy of *My Goals #1*. Write the word *listening* where everyone can see it. Ask students how many of them think listening actively is an easy goal to achieve. Explain that there are several skills involved in being effective listeners just as there are several skills involved with being a good softball player.

2. Explain that, just as a softball player wants to concentrate and practice the skills needed to improve, students need to identify the listening skills they could improve. Discuss situations where students feel they could be better listeners at school, at home, and in the community and have them write these goals on their goal sheet. Some example goals are: paying closer attention in class, keeping from being distracted, or following a coach's directions.

CLOSURE

Summarize the lesson, review its relevance to students, and tie it to future learning. Say to the students,

> *We have set an important goal and next time we will begin working on the first skill to achieve our listening goal. By signing and dating your goal sheet, you are promising to concentrate and work on your goal. I will sign your goal sheets meaning I will help you reach your goals. The third line is for your parent(s) to sign. Take this goal sheet home and tell your parents about your goal. You can teach them all about listening as you learn new skills! Bring your goal sheets back by ___.*

HINT

Offer a tangible or social reward for returning the goal sheet. Keep the goal sheet in each student's portfolio.

My Goals #1

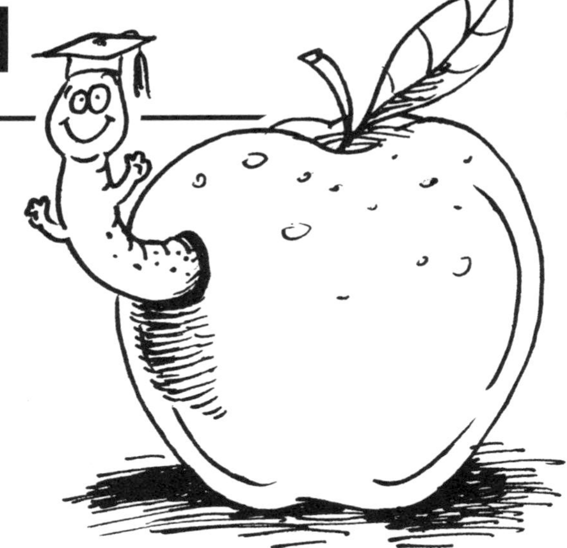

My goal is ______________________________

____

____

At home, I will ____

____

At school, I will ____

____

In my community, I will ____

____

Name: ______________________________ Date: ____________________

Family Member: ______________________ Date: ____________________

Teacher: ____________________________ Date: ____________________

GIVE ME FIVE: LISTENING

GOAL

To improve listening skills

BACKGROUND INFORMATION

The *Give Me Five* strategy addresses listening versus hearing, use of body posture, and key phrases to signal the need to listen. The main focus of this lesson is to provide students with a strategy that helps them be prepared and attentive for the task of listening. We all "drop out" of listening situations from time to time but if we don't bring ourselves back, we can lose track of what is being said. The *Give Me Five* strategy can be used by educators to bring students to attention and it can help students bring themselves back to a listening situation.

Be aware of the misconception that good listeners keep their eyes focused on the speaker at all times (Jalongo, 1991). Although the *Give Me Five* strategy does ask students to keep their eyes on the speaker, the strategy is used to focus attention rather than to expect that students will maintain eye contact throughout the listening situation. Also be aware that expectations for listening behaviors may differ in various cultures.

OBJECTIVES

1. Tell the difference between listening and hearing.
2. Be aware of the importance of listening versus hearing to gain knowledge.
3. Use an appropriate listening position: eyes on the speaker, mouth quiet, body still, ears listening, and hands free.
4. Listen for specific information.

MATERIALS

1. *Give Me Five* graphic (See page 28; duplicate and enlarge the graphic, color it, mount it onto poster board, and laminate it for durability, if desired.)

2. *Barn Dance!* (1986) by Bill Martin Jr. and John Archambault (If desired, substitute another book. It is preferable that the book have sound words or objects that might make sounds. It is more enjoyable if the sound words do not match the expected sound source [e.g., in this story, the owl speaks, the wind "plinks" on a violin, the crow calls a square dance, and the male character is a "tickin' and a tockin'" as he dances.)

INTRODUCTION

Tie-in to Prior Learning

Refer to the goal-setting activity from the previous lesson. The students wrote goals addressing listening at school, at home, and in the community. Review their goals.

Focus/Relevancy

1. Ask the students what they think of when they hear the phrase "give me five." Discuss slapping hands to celebrate someone doing a good job on something, or teammates giving a "high five" to each other when the team scores a point. Say to the students,

   We are going to use "give me five" in a different way. We are going to use this phrase as a tool to remind us about listening. How do you think the phrase "give me five" could help us listen?

2. Have students brainstorm responses. At this point in the lesson, students will not know the answer but this will start them thinking. Explain that they will be learning about what *listening effectively* means using a new kind of "give me five" to remind them of the body language necessary to listen. Discuss with students how the *Give Me Five* strategy could help them be better prepared to listen. Explain that they will be learning about what body language they can use to help them be better listeners.

3. Brainstorm the importance of listening (e.g., listening is important for safety reasons, gathering information, playing games, telling jokes, enjoying music). Brainstorm the consequences for not listening (e.g., not understanding a joke, not knowing the rules of the game, getting in trouble). Stress that by practicing the *Give Me Five* strategy, students will be taking the first steps to being better listeners, being prepared to listen, and being focused throughout a lesson.

LESSON ACTIVITIES

1. Discuss with students the difference between hearing and listening. Explain that there are sounds around us constantly but we may not be aware of them. Have the students sit quietly for a few moments to listen and identify some of the sounds. Pause to listen. Ask the students what was different when they paused to listen. Explain that the sounds around them were there all along but until their brains were engaged as listeners they were not always aware of them, so the sounds had no meaning. To listen for meaning, the brain has to be engaged.

2. Share your observations of how during step 1, when the students were pausing to listen, their "body language" showed that their brains were engaged and listening was taking place. Give examples of the different styles of listening posture that were exhibited (e.g., everyone was still, everyone was

quiet, some students were looking down while others looked at the teacher or around the room). An enjoyable way to explore "body language" is to role-play various scenarios. For example, have students slouch in their seats as if they are bored. Have students show their feelings through their body language. Then have them pretend that someone has brought in a tray of cupcakes and contrast that scenario with someone bringing in a tray of rotten fruit. Allow time for students to respond and then discuss messages that can be sent through body language.

3. Show the *Give Me Five* poster showing the gesture of an outstretched palm. Discuss what each of the five fingers means (i.e., eyes on the speaker, mouth quiet, body still, ears listening, and hands free). One way to explain each of the *Give Me Five* fingers is through role-playing. The following are suggestions for role-playing:

   - *Eyes on the speaker*—Discuss that the speaker may not always be a teacher. The speaker is whoever is talking and could be another student, a parent, a visitor, or a friend; and listening rules still apply. Practice having students use this strategy while listening to a poem or short story. Discuss what helps them remember information best. Once the students know the listening task, it may no longer be necessary to keep their eyes continually on the speaker, although it may help to keep them focused on the information being given.

   - *Mouth quiet*—Role-play students returning from recess. After signalling "give me five," compliment students on how quickly they demonstrated listening posture. Discuss that during some listening tasks, the listener may think of events to share, but may have to wait until a later time to share them. For example, if the student has a lot of knowledge about dinosaurs and the story is about Tyrannosaurus rex, he or she may have some expert information to share that will have to wait for another time. The story may make the student think about an exciting trip to a place having to do with dinosaurs, but once again, he or she has to wait for the right time to share the story.

   - *Body still*—Role-play by having the group twist or wiggle in their seats. After giving the "give me five" signal, have students stop all body movement and sit straight and tall in their seats. Discuss how body movements or posture affect how well the student and those around him or her listen. Have students demonstrate possible body positions appropriate for longer listening tasks (e.g., lying on the floor, standing beside their desks, or laying their heads on their desks). Note, however, that constantly changing from one position to another is distracting for the listener and those around him or her.

- *Ears listening*—Review the difference between simply hearing sounds and using the brain to identify the sound or message by listening. Role-play listening for the sounds at recess, the sounds of sleeping, or the sounds in a kitchen.

- *Hands free*—Have the entire group role-play cutting, writing, or being busy. When you hold up your hand and say "give me five," have the students stop what they are doing and put down their materials. (Students might fold their hands in their laps while listening or place their hands on their desks.) Role-play again. Have students pretend to listen to a story while being distracted by a really neat, new sports pencil. Have the students elicit ways to return to the listening task (e.g., putting the pencil away, purposely returning their attention to the speaker, extending their hands discretely in a "give me five" position).

4. Introduce the lesson's next listening task by discussing the importance of listening for the key words that teachers or speakers often use to signal an important message. When the students hear certain words or phrases, such as "give me five," "this is important," or "I hope you're listening carefully," students should immediately demonstrate an appropriate listening body position. Discuss that there will be times when the student will need to continue listening actively for extended periods of time. The students may have to give themselves a reminder to keep focused, just as in the role-playing examples when the students pretended to be distracted by a pencil and had to purposely ignore the distraction and return their attention to the speaker. To practice using the *Give Me Five* strategy during an activity that includes following directions in an extended listening task, read the book *Barn Dance!* (or the book chosen for this lesson). Remind the students that they will be using the *Give Me Five* strategy by demonstrating appropriate body language while listening. They should also discreetly use the "give me five" signal to help bring themselves back to the listening task if their attention wanders.

5. Discuss the author, illustrator, and any relevant vocabulary. (Note that steps 6–8 specifically address the book *Barn Dance!* Adapt as needed if a different story was chosen.) Before reading the book, highlight the literary components (see page 12). In addition, for the book *Barn Dance!* discuss the following:

   - Book cover—The cover depicts a barn with a scarecrow and various farm animals. After showing the cover of the book, ask the students if they think the setting is an urban or rural area. What clues did they use?

   - Setting—The first illustration is of a farmhouse and field, which is brightly lit by the moon. Ask the students what time of day they think it is. How can they tell? Why is it so bright?

6. Introduce the listening task in which the students are going to signal with a "thumbs up" when they hear the following sound words or sound sources:

   a. the owl (Have students predict what the owl might say.)

   b. plink, plink, plink (Have students guess what might be making this sound.)

   c. tickin' and tockin' (Also have students predict what might make this sound.)

   (These sound words are specific examples from the *Barn Dance!* book. If substituting another book, look for specific words that the students must listen for.) Restate the listening job and model the signal with the students as you review the sound words.

7. Read the story. As each sound word is read, praise students' active listening as indicated by the "thumbs up." If students appear to lose concentration while listening, model a "give me five" signal to bring them back to the listening task. While reading, point out the following literary highlights:

   - Setting—Note the boy listening at the window. Predict sounds he might hear on a still night in the country. Contrast with city sounds at night.
   - Vocabulary—Ask students what a *hoedown* is. Talk about the kind of dancing that is done at a hoedown. (Students may also call it a *square dance*.)
   - Phonological awareness—Note the rhythm of the story. Does it sound like a rap?

8. After reading the story, discuss how the "plink, plink, plink" and "tickin' and tockin'" sounds were used in the story. Were the students' predictions accurate? Point out the following literary highlights:

   - Vocabulary—Discuss or clarify the meaning of the following words as used in this story: *curtsey, bow, twilight, dawn, sunrise, dusk, evening,* and *sunset*.
   - Real versus fiction—Discuss real versus pretend. The story has animals that attend a dance in the barn. Ask the students if they think this story could really have happened.
   - Similes—Discuss what the author might have meant by the following expressions: *music honeyed up, there's magic in the air..., as quiet as a feather on a breath of air....*" Ask the students if they think anyone heard the boy as he went up the stairs. Expand on the effectiveness of the author in using this kind of expression.
   - Illustrations—Discuss the use of color to show warm oranges as the sun comes up and cool purples and blues to show night.

9. Ask students to discuss how they used the *Give Me Five* strategy to maintain appropriate body language for listening throughout the story. Did the strategy help to maintain their focus?

CLOSURE

Summarize the lesson, review its relevance to students, and tie it to future learning. Have students tell why it is important to be prepared for listening and review the *Give Me Five* strategy. Discuss other classroom situations or home situations where appropriate body language is beneficial for a listening task (e.g., listening for safety information, listening to a parent about where to meet after school). As an educator, use this new strategy throughout the day as a way to gain students' attention (e.g., when students line up for lunch or recess, when giving instructions, when giving important information pertaining to assignments and / or homework).

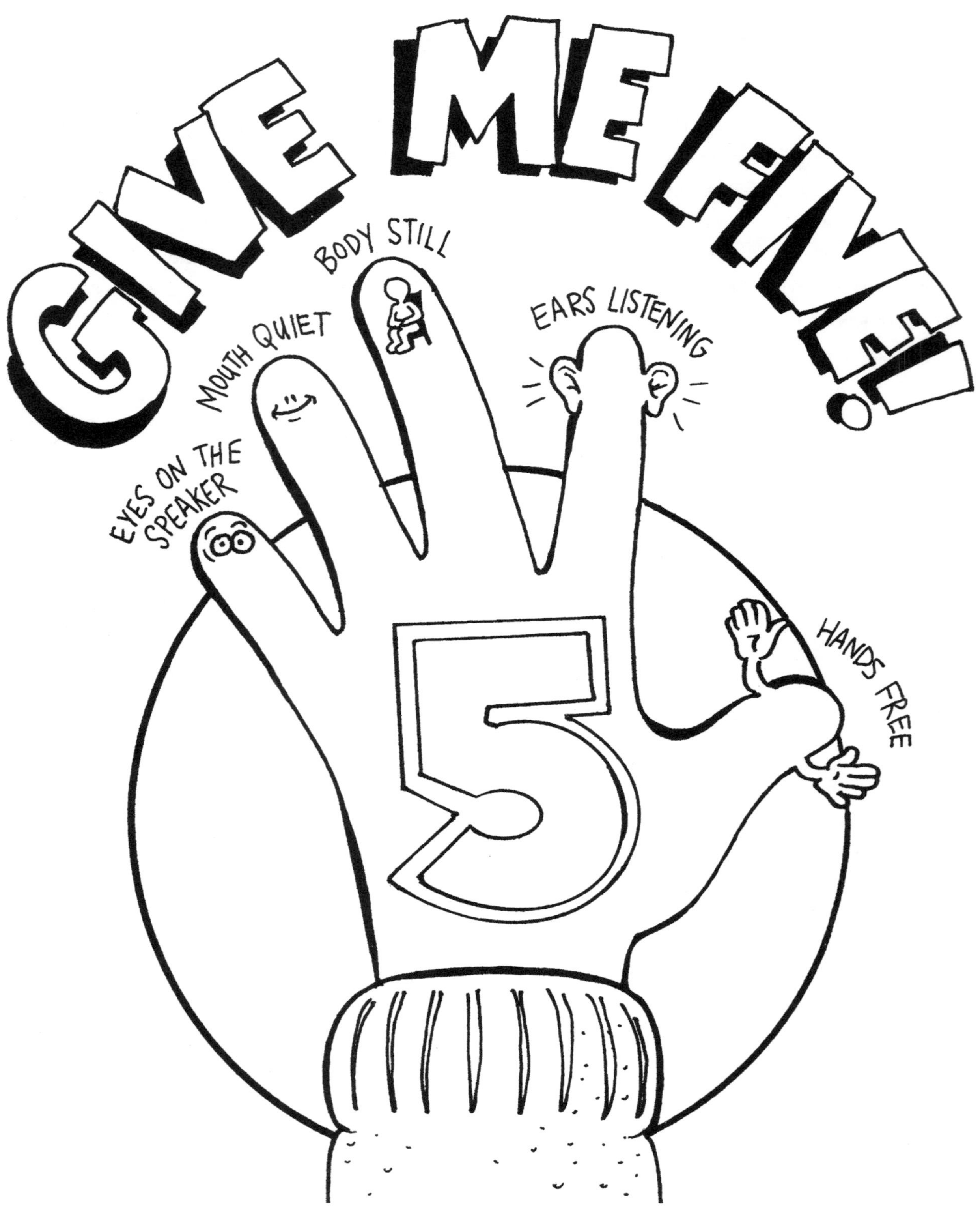
GIVE ME FIVE!
EYES ON THE SPEAKER
MOUTH QUIET
BODY STILL
EARS LISTENING
HANDS FREE
5

CARE: LISTENING (PART I)

GOAL

To improve listening skills

BACKGROUND INFORMATION

The main focus of the *CARE* strategy, Parts I and II, is to provide students with an opportunity to listen actively for extended periods of time with the addition of distractors. The distractors in this lesson are both physical (props) and environmental (neighbors with props, a variety of speakers, frequent group responses, and sound effects). The distractions are presented in an activity that has students produce a radio show.

In these lessons, an analogy is made between static on a radio (i.e., when too many signals distract from the main signal) and the disruption to listening (i.e., when there are too many distractions in the students' listening environment). Students are helped to recognize listening distractions and to "tune them out" by practicing the *CARE* strategy (i.e., concentrating on the listening job, alerting the brain when key words signal the need to listen, repeating the important information silently, and evaluating the information to ensure understanding). They are also taught to "tune in" the appropriate auditory message. It is recommended that both lessons be reviewed before teaching Part I.

OBJECTIVES

1. Listen actively for specific information.
2. Identify interfering noises or distractions.
3. Recognize the need for clarification.

MATERIALS

1. A radio
2. *CARE* graphic (See page 33; duplicate and enlarge the graphic, color it, mount it onto poster board, and laminate it for durability, if desired.)
3. *Possum Come a-Knockin'* (1990) by Nancy Van Laan (If desired, substitute another book. *Possum Come a-Knockin'* was selected because of its use of a variety of entertaining characters who are all involved in some type of activity which lends itself to a sound effect [e.g., "Granny was a sittin' and a rockin' and a knittin'; Ma was busy cookin' in the kitchen makin' taters"]. Any book that uses repetitive patterns and action will work.)

INTRODUCTION

Tie-in to Prior Learning

Remind students that in the previous lesson, they listened and watched for the *Give Me Five* strategy to prepare for listening actively. A listener who is listening actively makes sure that his or her brain is engaged in listening rather than just *hearing words that may have no meaning*. The listener's body language shows that he or she is prepared to listen. In this lesson, the students will practice "tuning out" distractions or static in order to have a clear signal. The analogy is made to a radio show. The listening job in this lesson will be a little more difficult because there will be added distractions and the listening task extends for a period of time.

Focus/Relevancy

1. Turn on the radio and use it to demonstrate static. Tune a radio station so that the music can barely be heard because of the static. Discuss what is wrong with the music signal. Explain that the music is the desired signal, but that there is more than one signal coming in at the same time. These unwanted signals cause static.

2. Discuss why it is not very pleasant to listen to music this way. Ask what is needed to improve the quality of the signal. Encourage the idea of "tuning in to one signal" to make it clearer. Demonstrate this point by tuning the radio to a clear signal. With students, brainstorm situations at school, at home, or in other places where they have had distractions (e.g., the classroom when there is noise from other classes, at home studying for a test when younger siblings are bothersome, at the movies when someone close by is talking too loudly, during class when feeling hungry or when thinking about what to do after school).

3. Ask students why it is important to listen even when they are distracted. Elicit consequences for not listening for the situations brainstormed by students in step 2. Discuss ways to avoid these problems by "tuning out distractions" and "tuning into one clear signal" (e.g., moving away from the noise source, ignoring the noise, concentrating harder, making sure to eat a good breakfast, etc.).

LESSON ACTIVITIES

1. Show the *CARE* poster and explain the acronym CARE:

   - *Concentrate*—Discuss the need to be "tuned in," which requires effort on the part of the listener.

   - *Alert your brain*—Discuss how the use of key words, such as "Give me five," or "This is important" signal that it is time to listen.

- *Repeat silently*—Discuss how the skill of repeating information or directions silently can help the listener remember the information. For example, when given directions to a location such as a post office, one might repeat the directions silently until information can be written down or until you get to the location.

- *Explain or evaluate*—Discuss the need to check for understanding. Does the message make sense? Point out the polka-dotted elephant on the poster. A polka-dotted elephant does not make sense; it needs clarification. Is the message clear or is the message a "polka-dotted elephant"? Is there a need to request clarification? Say to the students,

  When we do not understand what the speaker is saying, it is like the static on the radio. When the message is unclear, it needs to be fine-tuned. We can ask for clarification to make sure that we understand the message. Do you hear the little word clarify *in this big word?* (Use the golf clap [see page 13] to clap the syllables while saying the word *clar/i/fi/ca/tion* together.)

  Model asking for clarification. Encourage students to ask for more information when needed and suggest students begin to use this strategy independently.

2. Tell the students they are going to listen to a story that will become the script for a radio show that they will perform. The book is called *Possum Come a-Knockin'*. Tell the students that their first listening job will be to signal each time they hear a new character mentioned. Ask students if they are ready to listen.

   If the students assume that they are ready to follow the directions without requesting clarification, prompt with questions such as, "Who would like to demonstrate how we will signal? When are we supposed to signal? What is a 'new' character?" Because the goal is to have students recognize the need for clarification, these details are purposely not explained. If necessary, ask, "Does anyone need clarification?" Allow time for students to ask additional questions (i.e., concerning specifics of the instructions, what a character is, what the signal will be, etc.). Explain the term *character* if necessary.

3. Students are to signal a "thumbs up" each time they hear a new character mentioned as the story is read. To check for understanding, practice following the directions with the first page of the story.

4. Before reading the story, highlight the literary components (see page 12). Discuss the author and illustrator. In addition, highlight the following:

   - Cover—Ask students to describe the possum character illustrated (e.g., sneaky, mischievous).

   - Setting—Ask students if they think this story is written about someone who lives in a large city.

Discuss and note how the dialect, illustrations, and writing style depict a rural setting.

5. While reading the story, point out the following literary highlights:
   - Vocabulary—Define some of the words used by the author: *cookin', knockin', rockin', knittin', taters, whittlin', twiny, winder, scoot, pappy,* and *granny.* Discuss how the author has used this style of writing to set the mood for the story.
6. After reading the story, point out the following literary highlights:
   - Similes—Have students explain how Possum *made a fool out of me.*
   - Real versus fiction—Discuss whether this story is real or pretend. How do students know?

CLOSURE

Summarize the lesson, repeat its relevance to students, and tie it to future learning. After reading the story, talk about how the students actively listened by signaling with a "thumbs up." Ask if there were any distractions that had to be "tuned out" or ignored. Have students describe one other distracting situation where the *CARE* strategy could be applied.

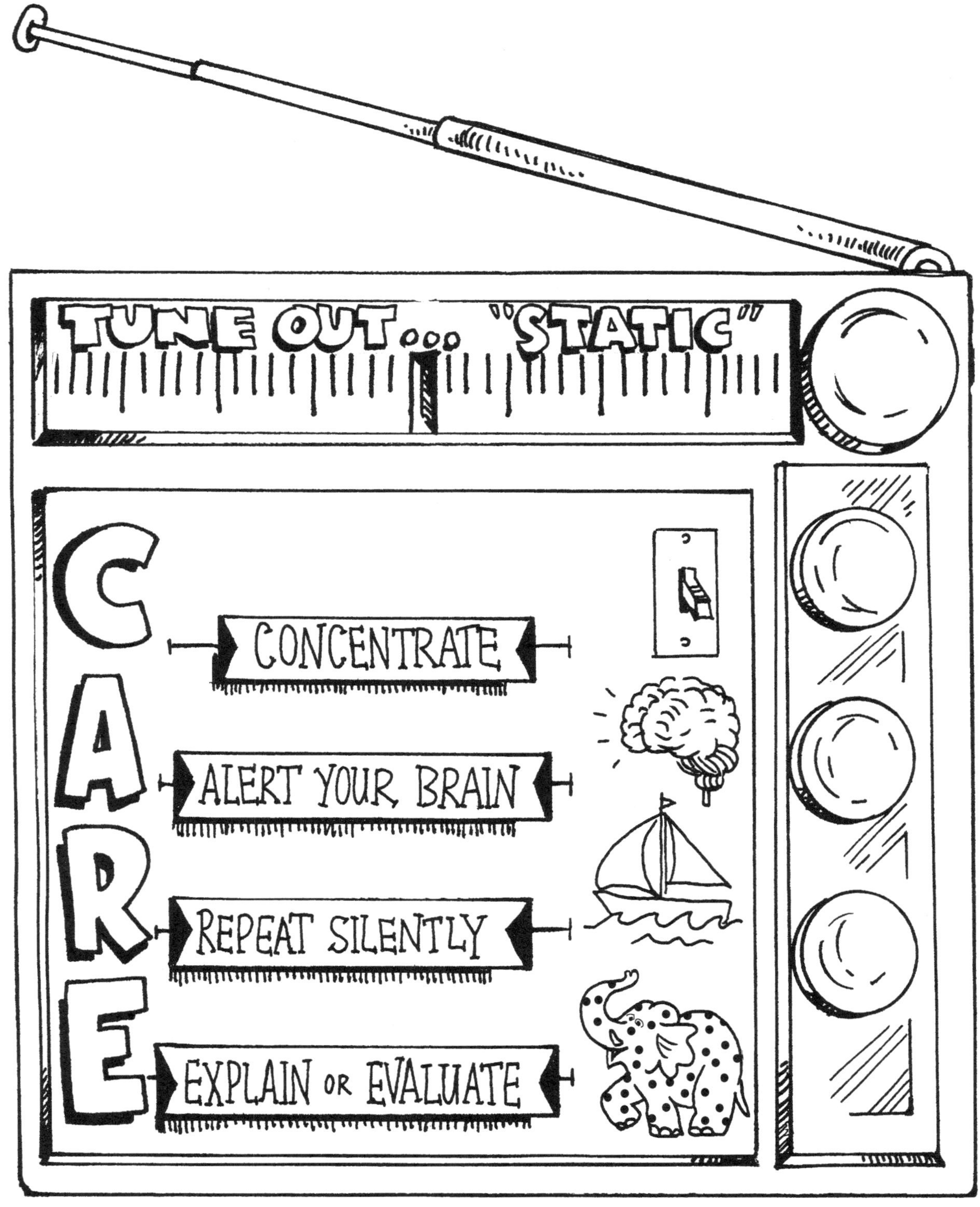
TUNE OUT... "STATIC"
C
A
R
E
CONCENTRATE
ALERT YOUR BRAIN
REPEAT SILENTLY
EXPLAIN OR EVALUATE

CARE: LISTENING (PART II)

GOAL

To improve listening skills

BACKGROUND INFORMATION

The main focus of the *CARE* strategy, Parts I and II, is to provide students with an opportunity to listen actively for extended periods of time with the addition of distractors. The distractors in this lesson are both physical (props) and environmental (neighbors with props, a variety of speakers, frequent group responses, and sound effects) which are included in a radio show. It is recommended that both lessons be reviewed before teaching them.

In these lessons, an analogy is made between static on a radio (i.e., when too many signals distract from the main signal) and the disruption to listening (i.e., when there are too many distractions in the students' listening environment). Students are helped to recognize listening distractions, to "tune them out" by practicing the *CARE* strategy (i.e., concentrating on the listening job, alerting the brain when key words signal the need to listen, repeating the important information silently, and evaluating the information to ensure understanding), and to "tune in" the appropriate auditory message.

In Part II, students make a radio show by following a script. It is helpful for younger readers or nonreaders if all parts are read by the educator and the students respond with sound effects and gestures when it's their characters' turn. It is helpful for students with reading difficulties if all parts are read together as a group before enacting the radio show. The amount of time needed for the session could be reduced by having the educator take the role of the narrator. Part II activities may take several 30-minute sessions to complete.

OBJECTIVES

1. Tune in to an auditory cue and respond by performing an action.
2. Tune out distractions.

MATERIALS

1. *CARE* poster (Created earlier)
2. *The Possum Script* (See pages 38–41; duplicate one per student. Or create a script for the story that was read in Part I.)
3. Tape recorder and cassette tape or video recording equipment
4. Sound effect instruments (e.g., tongue depressors or popsicle sticks for knitting needles, rubber bands on facial-tissue boxes or plastic butter tubs for twiny line, ribbed sticks for whittlin', tone

blocks or sticks from the music room for bangin', paper cups and plastic forks for stirrin', sandpaper blocks, scratch rug, or fabric for dog scratchin')

INTRODUCTION

Tie-in to Prior Learning

Remind students that in the last lesson they read the story *Possum Come a-Knockin'* and identified the different characters. They had to practice being CAREful listeners! Review the *CARE* poster.

Focus/Relevancy

1. Ask students how a radio is like a TV and how are they different. Discussion could include the fact that radio relies on sounds to tell a story rather than visual pictures. The listener has to rely on his or her sense of hearing rather than his or her sense of sight. Radio programs often use sound effects to make the story seem more real.

2. Through class discussion, review the importance of listening in distracting situations. Have students brainstorm distracting situations for them (e.g., a brother listening to loud music when you're on the telephone, friends laughing when announcements are being made by your teacher). Review the consequences for not listening in each situation brainstormed. Review ways to avoid these problems by tuning out distractions and tuning into one clear signal (e.g., moving away from the noise source, applying the *Give Me Five* strategy, applying the *CARE* strategy [i.e., making yourself concentrate, alerting your brain, repeating the information silently, and asking questions for clarification]).

LESSON ACTIVITIES

1. The students are now ready to make a radio show. Explain to students that their program will be recorded and that any noises made with instruments, scripts, or voices will be picked up by the recorder. Remind the students that these noises will create static for the listener. Tell them,

   You will be playing a character, or a part, from the story and each character will have a sound effect that goes with the action he or she is doing. Some of the sound effects will be made with instruments or objects and some can be made easily with your own voices. It is very important to be tuned in so you will know when it's your turn to make the sound effect. When you hear your character's name it will be your cue to make your sound effect.

   Discuss that a *cue* is a signal to let the students know when it's their turn to perform their sound effect. Explain that their cues for the radio show will be the names of their characters. When they hear their character's name, they need to be ready to say their parts and perform their sound effect. Remind students of the *CARE* strategy.

2. Pass out *The Possum Script* and assign character parts. (Note that the script is not identical to the book but still honors the cadence of the sentences. The script is written with first-person pronouns to increase the involvement of students. Also, words are written as children more commonly see them [e.g., *rocking* rather than *rockin'*] but the endings can be dropped when the scripts are read, if desired.) Assign as many students as you wish for each part. Practice reading through the script and discuss: inflection for questions (vocal pitch goes up) and answers (vocal pitch goes down), the dialogue, characterization through voice, the role of the narrator, and how to follow and read a script. The characters and/or sound effects are as follows:

   - Narrator—reads the bold print and draws out the word *when* (i.e., *wheeeen*).
   - Granny—uses tongue depressors or popsicle sticks to make the sound of knitting.
   - Ma—uses paper cups and plastic spoons to make a stirring sound.
   - Pa—uses tone blocks or sticks to bang or pound.
   - Pappy—uses two sticks to make a whittling sound.
   - Sister—makes a happy or fussy baby sound.
   - Brother—uses rubber bands on a facial-tissue box or a butter tub to sound like untangling twiny line.
   - Tom-cat—makes a hissing sound.
   - Coon-dawg—howls and uses fabric for scratching sound.
   - Possum—knocks twice on a table or something wooden.

   Point out that the narrator reads the bold print and the characters read only their part followed by the sound effect. (If necessary, use a colored marker to highlight the parts of each student. But remember this is primarily a listening task; it is more important that students listen for their cue than to know the dialogue perfectly.) Practice having the narrator draw out the word "wheeeen" and all students following with, "Possum came a-knocking on my door." Once all students know their parts, tell them they are ready to begin the radio show.

3. Pass out the sound effect instruments randomly. **No time to panic but you just handed noise-makers to a classroom full of children!!** Stress to the children (or have another adult help with

noise control) that as you are passing out the instruments, they are challenged to keep them on their desks (or on the floor if seated on the floor) until it is their turn to make a sound effect. Rehearse making each sound effect for a short period of time after each character reads his or her line. Direct students to stop making the sound effect when the narrator reads, "Wheeeen." Remember, the class follows with, "Possum came a-knocking on my door."

4. Tape-record the radio show. Make sure that the tape recorder is placed where it can pick up all sound effects. Add a fun, professional recording atmosphere by saying,

   Quiet on the set! 5..., 4..., 3..., 2..., 1..., presenting the Reader Theater Radio Show's production of Nancy Van Laan's, Possum Come a-Knockin', *starring (Mrs. Jones second-grade class).*

   Have the narrator begin. Continue recording until the radio show is completed. Collect the instruments while rewinding the tape for listening.

5. Have the class listen and evaluate their performance and the accuracy of their sound effects. Ask,

   Were there many distracting sounds? Does it take a lot of effort to concentrate for a performance? How does this performance compare with how you have to perform each day in the classroom with distractions all around you? What helped you concentrate with all these distractions?

6. Have the class repeat this experience to improve their listening or just for fun.

CLOSURE

Summarize the lesson, review its relevance to students, and tie it to future learning. Remind the students that they have been listening actively for cues while tuning out any distractions or static. They have had to concentrate, alert their brains to listen for cues, repeat the directions silently in their minds, remember what to do when it was their cue, and evaluate how they completed their parts in order to improve with each turn. The students also evaluated the directions they had to follow as they learned to read a script and plan the taping of their show.

In the next lesson, the students will be practicing what to do when they have evaluated directions that don't make sense.

The Possum Script

Characters:	Narrator	Granny	Ma	Pa	Pappy
	Sister	Brother	Coon-dawg	Tom-cat	Possum

Narrator: **Possum came a-knocking on my door, on my door.**
Possum came a-knocking on my door.
Granny said...

Granny: I'm just a-sitting and a-rocking and a-knitting...

Narrator: **Wheeeen...**

All: Possum came a-knocking on my door.

Possum: [*Knocks twice*]

Narrator: **Ma said...**

Ma: I'm just busy cooking in the kitchen making taters...

Narrator: **Wheeeen...**

All: Possum came a-knocking on my door.

Possum: [*Knocks twice*]

Narrator: **Pa said...**

Pa: I'm just busy fixing and a-banging and a-pounding...

Narrator: **Wheeeen...**

All: Possum came a-knocking on my door.

Possum: [*Knocks twice*]

Narrator: **Pappy said...**

Pappy: I'm just a-whittling,
making play toys for the baby.

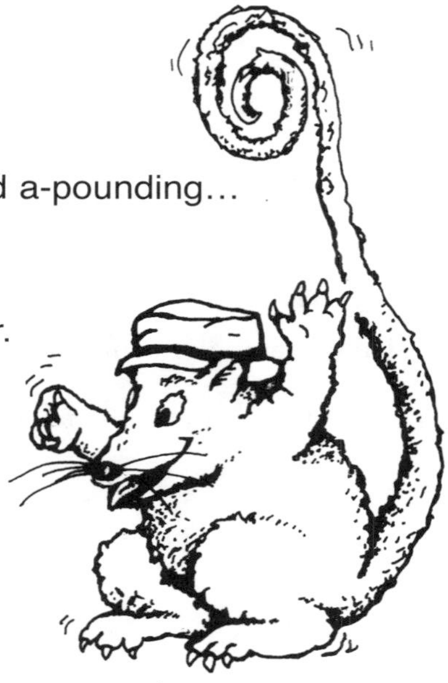

Narrator: **Wheeeen...**

All: Possum came a-knocking on my door.

Possum: [*Knocks twice*]

Narrator: **Sister said...**

Sister: I'm just tossing Baby up
while Pappy is a-whittling...

Narrator: **Wheeeen...**

All: Possum came a-knocking on my door.

Possum: [*Knocks twice*]

Narrator: **Brother said...**

Brother: I'm just untangling all the twiny line for fishing
while Sister's tossing Baby
and Pappy is a-whittling and Pa is busy fixing
and Ma is busy cooking and Granny is a-knitting...

Narrator: **Wheeeen...**

All: Possum came a-knocking on my door.

Possum: [*Knocks twice*]

Narrator: **Coon-dawg said...**

Coon-dawg: I'm just a-twitching and a-scratching in my corner...

Narrator: **Wheeeen...**

All: Possum came a-knocking on my door.

Possum: [*Knocks twice*]

Narrator: **Tom-cat said...**

Tom-cat: I'm just a-sniffing and a-spitting and a-hissing...

Narrator: **Wheeeen...**

All: Possum came a-knocking on my door.

Sister: What's that?

Brother: I don't know!

Granny: But that cat ought to go.

Narrator: **Then Coon-dawg started sniffing…**

Coon-dawg: And I'm pawing and a-growling.

Narrator: **While the Tom-cat, tail a-twitching, said…**

Tom-cat: I'm a-hissing and a-howling.

Narrator: **And Granny stopped her knitting**
and Pappy stopped his whittling
and Baby started fussing
with Sis and Brother tussling
'cause Possum was a-knocking on the door.

All: Then I creeped across the floor and peeked outside the door.
It's Possum that's a-knocking on our door!

Possum: [*Knocks twice*]

Brother: I'm a-leaping!

Sister: I'm a-running!

Coon-dawg: I'm a-howling!

Pappy: I'm a-chuckling!

Granny: I'm a-twinkling!

Narrator: **And Ma followed Pa to the door.**

Pa: Now hush!

Ma: Now hush!

Pa: You all stop your hollering and your fussing and your tussling
'cause there's nothing that's a-knocking on our door.

Possum: [*Knocks twice*]

Pappy: No Possum?

Pa: No Possum.

All: Then we all started doing like before.
Granny was a-knitting.
And Pappy was a-whittling.
And Ma was a-cooking.
And Pa was a-fixing.
And Brother was untangling.
And Sister's tossing Baby.
And Coon-dawg was a-scratching.
And Tom-cat was a-licking.
And me? I'm just sitting and a-looking out the window
when I see what I see scoot up that old oak tree.

Possum was a-scooting and a-scrambling and a-dangling!
That Possum that was knocking made a fool out of me!

Narrator: **Wheeeen...**

All: Possum came a-knocking on my door.

Possum: [*Knocks twice*]

GIVE ME FIVE and CARE FOLLOW-UP ACTIVITIES

GOAL

To reinforce and review *Give Me Five* and *CARE* strategies

BACKGROUND INFORMATION

The main focus of this lesson is to review the previous two strategies. The strategy guide review pages will be compiled with similar pages into a booklet at the end of the school year. This booklet, along with a vacation calendar, provide a means of practicing with family members and reinforcing skills throughout a school break. Although some educators may choose to do the strategy guide pages and homework activities at the end of each lesson, others prefer delayed reinforcement to strengthen knowledge of strategies, concepts, and vocabulary covered within the lessons. Using a small representation of the strategy poster, the strategy guide pages include the specific vocabulary from the lessons. An application component is provided on the second pages of the strategy guides. Students may do reflective writing about how the strategy is or can be useful to them.

OBJECTIVES

1. Tell and write the major components of the *Give Me Five* and *CARE* strategies.
2. Reflect and write about how the strategies will help at home, at school, and in the community.
3. Share strategy information with family members and complete the application activities.

MATERIALS

1. *Give Me Five* poster (Created earlier)
2. *CARE* poster (Created earlier)
3. *Give Me Five Strategy Guide* (See pages 44–45; duplicate one per student.)
4. *CARE Strategy Guide* (See pages 46–47; duplicate one per student.)
5. *Give Me Five Homework Activity* (See page 48; duplicate one per student.)
6. *CARE Homework Activity* (See page 49; duplicate one per student.)

INTRODUCTION

Tie-in to Prior Learning

Refer students to the initial goal-setting activity (see pages 19–20) and their completed goal sheets. Discuss that when setting their listening goals, they talked about some of the times and/or places that presented problems with listening actively and effectively. Point out that they have learned two strategies that will help them improve and move toward achieving their goals. Display the posters and review the *Give Me Five* and *CARE* strategies.

Focus/Relevancy

1. Introduce the idea of creating a *Strategy Guide Booklet* by saying,

   How many of you make lists that help you remember important things? We are going to be creating a special book throughout this year that will help you remember to be effective communicators in speaking, listening, and writing. The booklet will help you to remember all the strategies and skills you'll be learning this year.

2. Discuss how having the *Strategy Guide Booklet* will help them be more effective communicators at home, in school, and in the community. Explain that pages will be added as new strategies are learned and an entire booklet of strategies will be theirs to keep.

LESSON ACTIVITIES

1. Distribute the *Give Me Five Strategy Guid*e pages and the *CARE Strategy Guide* pages and have students complete the activities. Students should demonstrate they know the strategies by completing the blank lines. Point out to students that the choices are included on the page. Refer to the posters and have them displayed for the students.

2. On the second page of each strategy guide, have students write how each particular strategy has helped them or will help them at school, at home, or in the community. Brainstorm ideas (e.g., "I'll listen when the coach is talking at soccer practice," "I moved away from noise when it was important to listen to the teacher," "I picked a different seat to get away from the noisy popcorn muncher at the movie").

3. Hand out the *Give Me Five* and the *CARE Homework Activity* pages and discuss them. Reinforce the importance of sharing this information with family members, and the ease and fun of doing these assignments. They will only take a few minutes to complete, but students can impress their family with what they have learned! Have a reward system established to encourage students to bring their homework activity pages back to school signed by a family member.

CLOSURE

Summarize the lesson, review its relevance to students, and tie it to future learning. Discuss the objectives that were completed in this review (i.e., the students can tell and write the *Give Me Five* and *CARE* strategies; they can tell how they will use the strategies; they know the strategies well enough to share them with their family members). In the next lesson, the students will play a game that will exercise their communication skills while giving and following directions.

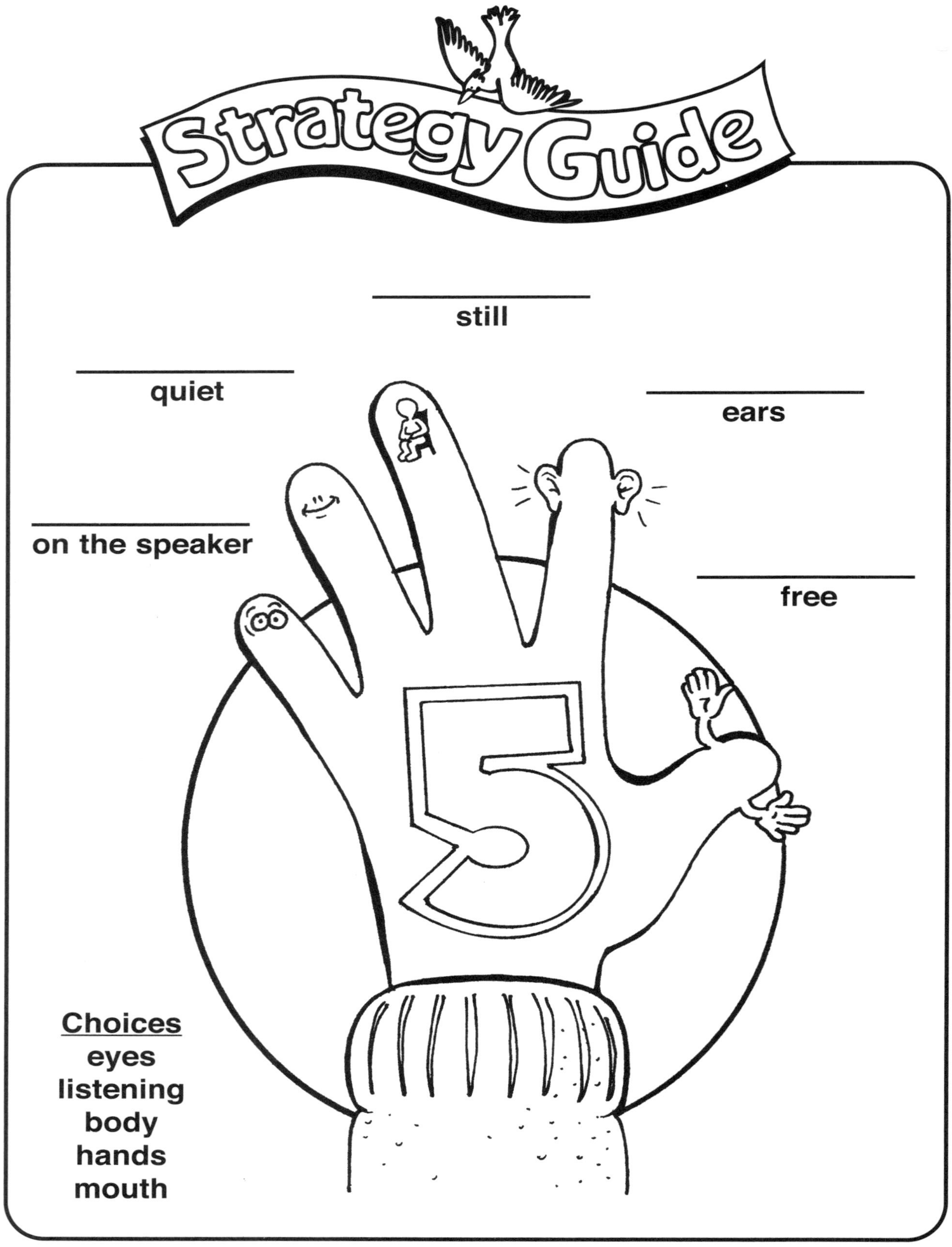
Strategy Guide
still
quiet
ears
on the speaker
free
5
Choices
eyes
listening
body
hands
mouth

Give Me Five: Listening

Name: ______________________________ Date: ______________

Directions: Write a sentence about how you have used or will use the strategy in each place.

At home, I ____

____

____

____

____

____

At school, I ____

____

____

____

____

____

In my community, I ____

____

____

____

____

____

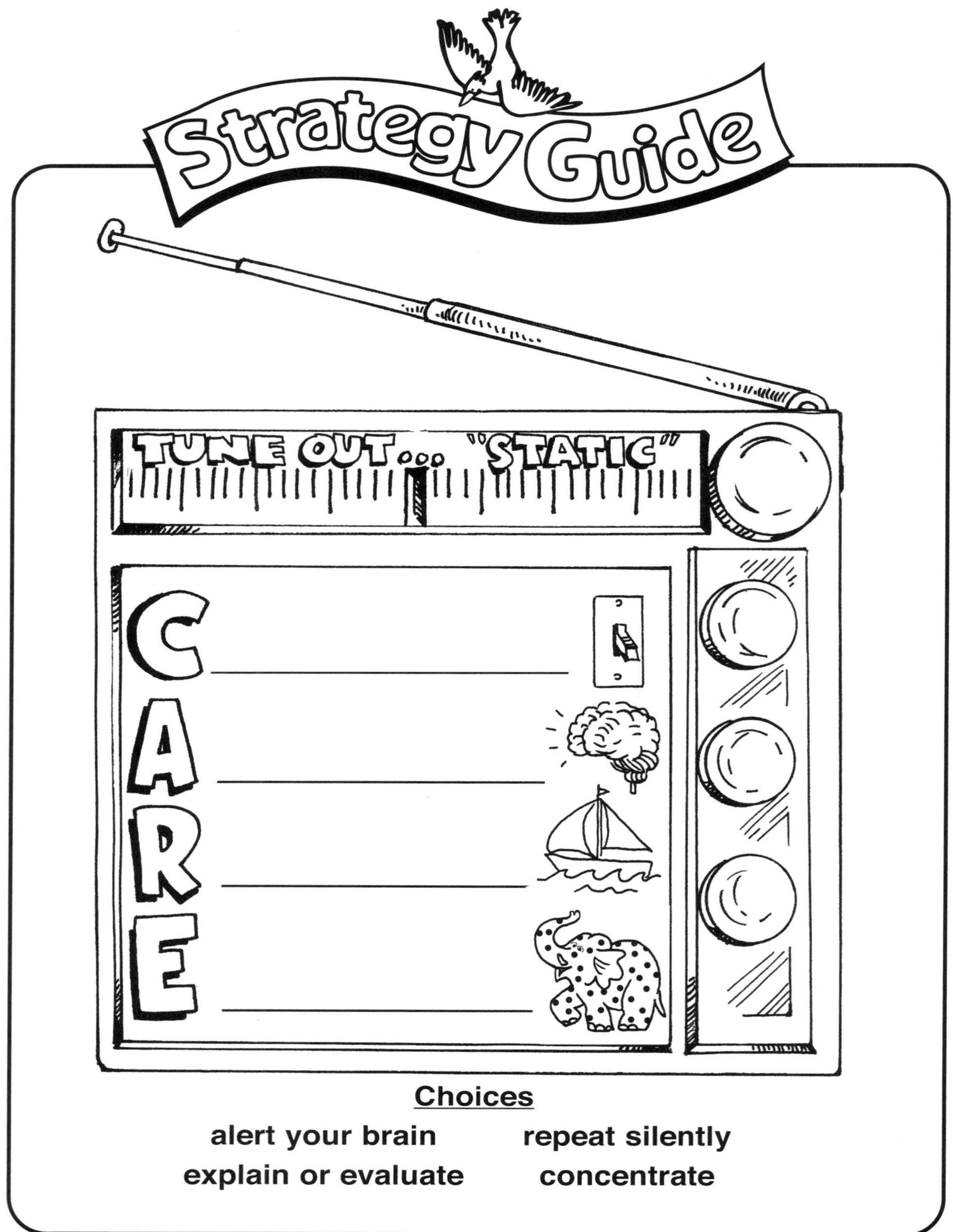
Strategy Guide
TUNE OUT... "STATIC"
C
A
R
E
Choices
alert your brain
repeat silently
explain or evaluate
concentrate

CARE: Listening

Name: ______________________________ Date: ______________

Directions: Write a sentence about how you have used or will use the strategy in each place.

At home, I ____

____

____

____

____

____

At school, I ____

____

____

____

____

____

In my community, I ______________________________________

____

____

____

____

____

Homework Activity

GIVE ME FIVE!
EYES ON THE SPEAKER
MOUTH QUIET
BODY STILL
EARS LISTENING
HANDS FREE
5

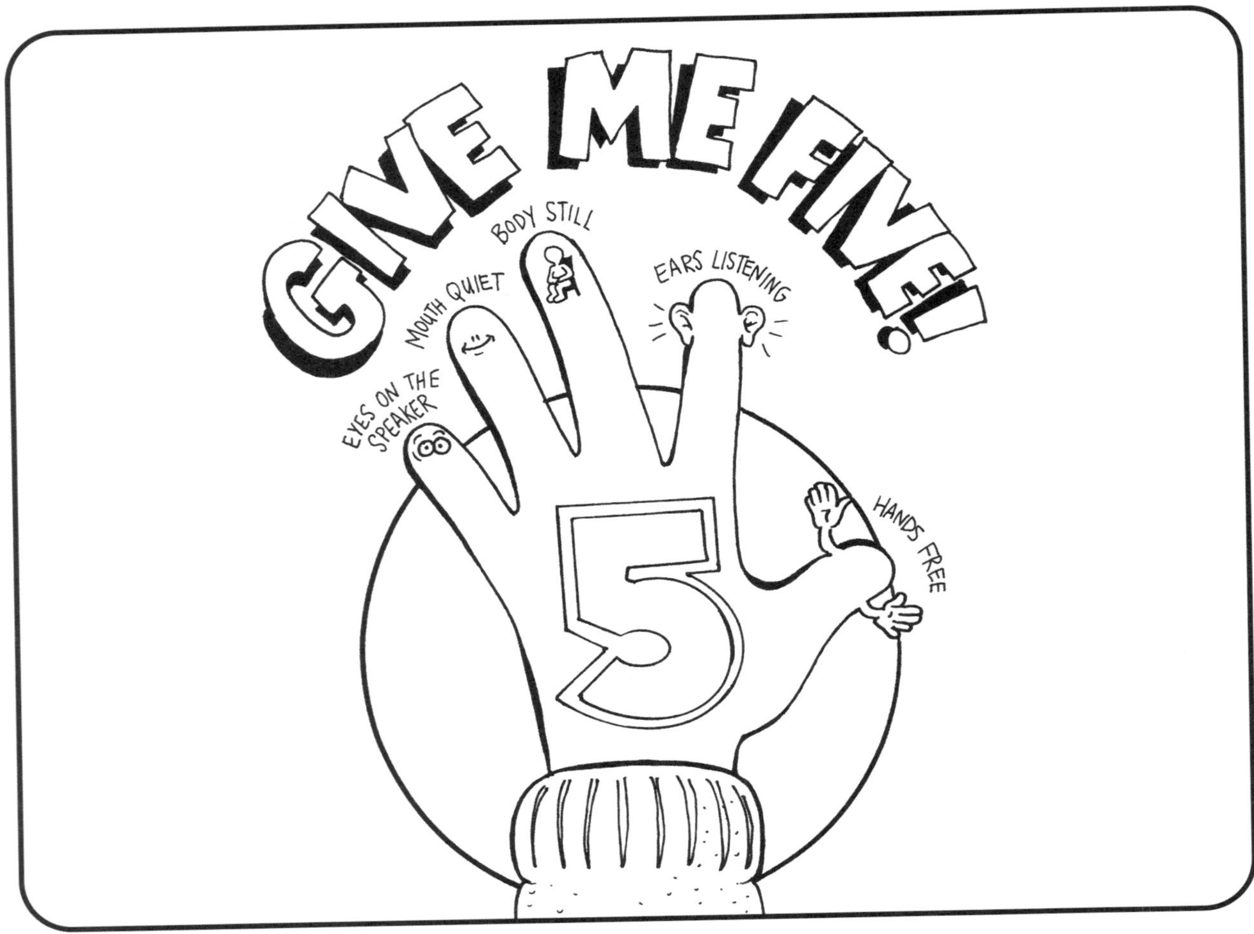

Dear Family,

1. Have your child explain the *Give Me Five* strategy and tell why it's important to listen actively.
2. Ask your child to name several situations where he or she could use the *Give Me Five* strategy. See how many places your child can name where listening is important.
3. Name a situation where listening is important. Ask your child to tell you the consequences for not listening in that situation.
4. If your child completes these activities, please sign below and return this form to school.

Family Member: ______________________________ Date: ______________

Homework Activity

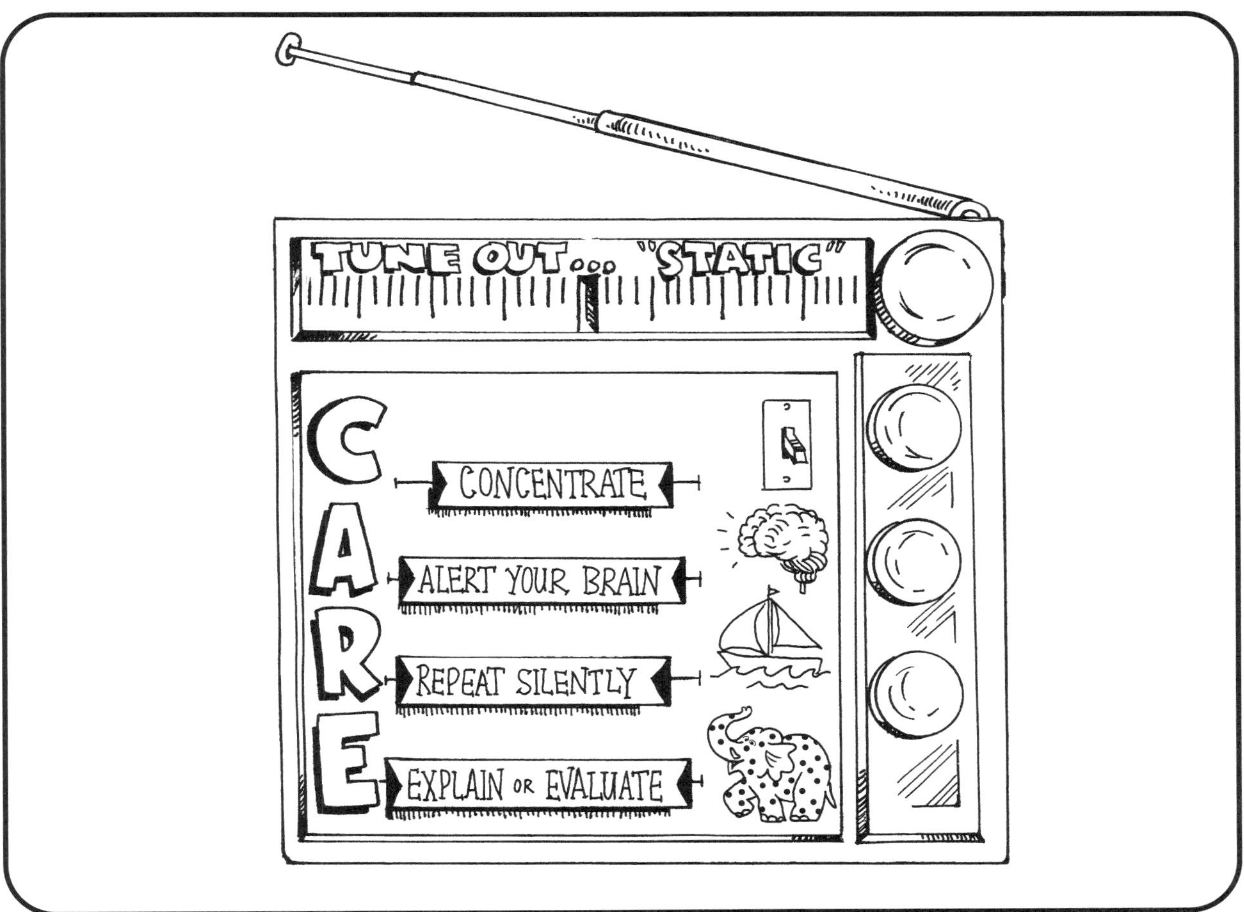

Dear Family,

1. There are distractions everywhere. It takes extra effort to listen under these conditions. Ask your child to explain the *CARE* strategy and how he or she can use it to be a better listener.
2. Have your child find the best places to do homework at your house. Ask where it is best to work when he or she really needs to concentrate on one thing. Have them tell why it's a good place to study.
3. Next time you're in a noisy grocery store, have your child practice *CARE*. Give him or her three items to remember and get for you.
4. If your child completes these activities, please sign below and return this form to school.

Family Member: ______________________________ Date: ______________

HIT THE BULL'S-EYE: GIVING AND RECEIVING DIRECTIONS

GOAL

To improve comprehension and oral expression skills

BACKGROUND INFORMATION

The main focus of this lesson is to evaluate given information. It encourages the student to ask the questions, "Does it make sense? Do I have enough information? Is it a reasonable request?" The educator should check out the "Hints" throughout the lesson which include shortcuts, variations, and helpful suggestions.

This lesson requires the use of barrier game boards and game pieces. Parent volunteers are wonderful for helping create the barrier games. Remember, these materials are reusable each year. A barrier game is one in which there is some type of barrier between the speaker and the listener so that they cannot see what the other person is doing. The barrier is removed after a direction is given and the listener and speaker analyze whether a communication breakdown occurred.

OBJECTIVES

1. Tell what the word *clarification* means.
2. Know when and how to ask for clarification when given insufficient directions or information by being an evaluative listener.

MATERIALS

1. *Hit the Bull's-Eye* graphic (See page 55; duplicate and enlarge the graphic, color it, mount it onto poster board, and laminate it for durability, if desired.)
2. Barrier game packets (Duplicate one packet per student. Create the game board by duplicating the two landscape pages [see pages 56–57] and gluing them onto a file folder. Color the landscape and laminate the file folder for durability. Duplicate the manipulable barrier game pieces [see pages 58–59]. Color, laminate, and cut them out. Place them in envelopes or individual plastic bags for each student.)

INTRODUCTION

Tie-in to Prior Learning

Review how to listen actively from the previous lesson when the students had to tune into the important information signal and tune out the static or distractions. Explain that the students are now ready to send and receive clear signals.

Focus/Relevancy

1. Directions need to be very specific to get a job done correctly. Discuss what might happen when information given to someone is not specific. For example, if birthday invitations were sent out that gave a street address but not a house number, few guests would attend or they might show up at the wrong house. The hosts would probably have a number of phone calls from friends asking for more information. Another example might be illustrated by asking the students what they would do if their teacher handed them the attendance sheet and asked them to take it to the office and give it to the President. Have students evaluate this request. Is it a reasonable or logical request? What if the teacher said, without pointing, "Give *this* to *that* teacher." Ask the students what the problem is with these directions. Do they know *exactly* what to do?

2. Show the *Hit the Bull's-Eye* poster. Read the questions on the poster to illustrate the lack of sufficient information from the examples (i.e., taking a note to the President, or giving the correct item to the correct person). Do students have enough information to follow the directions? Do the directions make sense? Do students need further clarification to make the directions clear? Ask the students how they would ask for clarification? Review what the word *clarification* means (i.e., discuss the clarity of the message). Refer to tuning in the signal and eliminating the static that keeps the message from coming in. Review the usefulness of questioning "polka-dotted elephant" messages. The goal is to follow or make a request clearly and concisely—straight to the bull's-eye!

LESSON ACTIVITIES

1. Pass out the barrier game packets and say to the students,

   I just put a lot of static on your desk! What do I mean by that?

   Discuss that static does not have to be verbal to be a distraction. Have the students use the *Give Me Five* strategy while they listen to these barrier game instructions,

   We will use these objects to play a listening game. In this game, you will be following directions to make your picture match another picture that you cannot see. You will have to listen very carefully so that you will know where to put the different pictures. We will try this game several times.

   The object of the first round is to lead the students to discover where communication can breakdown. Before selecting the student to give directions to the group, explain to the class that the person for the first round must be a risk-taker and that he or she will help the group learn by being the class "guinea pig."

2. Call on one student to give the first set of directions that the other students will be following. Set up a barrier or have the student move to a location where no one can see his or her map. Have that

student select four objects and quickly tape them on the barrier game board, so that he or she will be able to hold it up for the rest of the class to see after the first round of the game.

HINT

If a magnetic chalkboard is available, add magnetic strips to the game board and barrier game pieces. This allows everyone to see and to learn along with the student who is giving the directions.

3. Have the student give directions verbally for placement of the barrier game pieces. The others attempt to create the same arrangement with their game pieces as described. Explain that the listeners are not allowed to ask questions for clarification and must make "their best guesses" in placing their objects during round one.

4. The students are now ready to check for accuracy. Do not immediately show the direction-giver's barrier game board, which will be referred to as the key map. Explain to the class that it is important not to change their arrangement even if they do not match the key map. Have the direction-giver show the key map. Request a show of hands for matching arrangements. Analyze where any communication broke down. Was an unclear message given by the direction-giver or was the difference due to the listener?

HINT

Praise the students for their self-control and honesty as this round may not be very successful and the students are resisting the temptation to move their game pieces to match the key map.

5. For arrangements that did not match, analyze, as a group, the reasons for the differences. Ask the students what problems they encountered. Why didn't they hit the bull's-eye? What would need to be done differently to be more successful?

(Oftentimes, the direction-giver has not been specific enough in describing where the game pieces should be placed. But errors also occur because the listeners did not follow the direction appropriately. Be prepared for disagreement about who is at fault for the communication breakdown. Tape-record the next rounds of directions. The play back could help to settle the disagreements.)

Elicit discussion for each misplaced item. For example, if a tree was placed on the grass but it wasn't the tree intended by the direction-giver and it wasn't in the same position as the one on the key map, you could say,

If I asked you to put the tree on the grass, would you know which tree? There are three different types of trees to choose from. What could be said instead? There is also a large grassy area on your map. What direction could have been given to be more specific?

If the error was due to the listener, stress that students always want to be asking themselves the following questions:

- Does it make sense? Do I know the vocabulary?
- Do I need more information?
- Is it a reasonable request?

Explain that if the answer is no to any of these questions, they could follow one of the following steps:

- Ask for clarification—Model asking politely, "Excuse me, did you mean the pine tree, the pear tree, or the apple tree?" Stress that students need to use specific terms. Tell the students that in round two, they will be allowed to ask questions for clarification.

- Ask what a word means—It would not be specific enough to say, "Put the boat in the river" since there are pictures of both a sailboat and a rubber raft.

- Ask for more precise directions with reference points—Point out the compass to the students. Discuss the use of direction words such as north, south, east, west, to the right of, to the left of, above, below, on top, etc. Model giving directions such as, "Put the lake in the lower right-hand corner of the map," "Put the hill to the right of the lake above the rock."

6. Ask, "Now that you have the tools to 'Hit the Bull's-Eye' in giving and receiving directions, how many of you predict that by practicing your skills, you will greatly improve your accuracy the second time around?"

7. Select a new direction-giver and repeat the activity. Allow the students receiving directions to ask questions to clarify. Give assistance as needed by helping the direction-giver modify directions to be more specific. However, after comparing the direction-giver arrangement to the listeners' arrangements, a discussion of how the direction could have been stated differently usually has as much value in helping students be more specific in giving directions.

8. Check for success in matching arrangements by a show of hands, after the second round. If time allows, play another round as described above or divide into groups of two, taking turns having one person give and the second person follow the directions.

HINT

If dividing the group into pairs, give only a few minutes for placing the game pieces. Each pair could use folders as barriers or could be seated back-to-back. Have students use "six-inch voices" (see page 14) so that the noise level will stay low.

9. Practice for at least one more session with students who are having difficulty with this activity. Analyze where the difficulty occurs and review necessary concepts. Hold a discussion between each turn to find out whether the communication broke down and how communication could be improved.

CLOSURE

Summarize the lesson, review its relevance to students, and tie it to future learning. Ask the students why there were more matching arrangements after the second round. Why were they able to hit the bull's-eye more accurately? Remind students of the questions they should ask themselves when they are giving and receiving directions:

1. Does it make sense?
2. Do I need more information?
3. Is it a reasonable request?

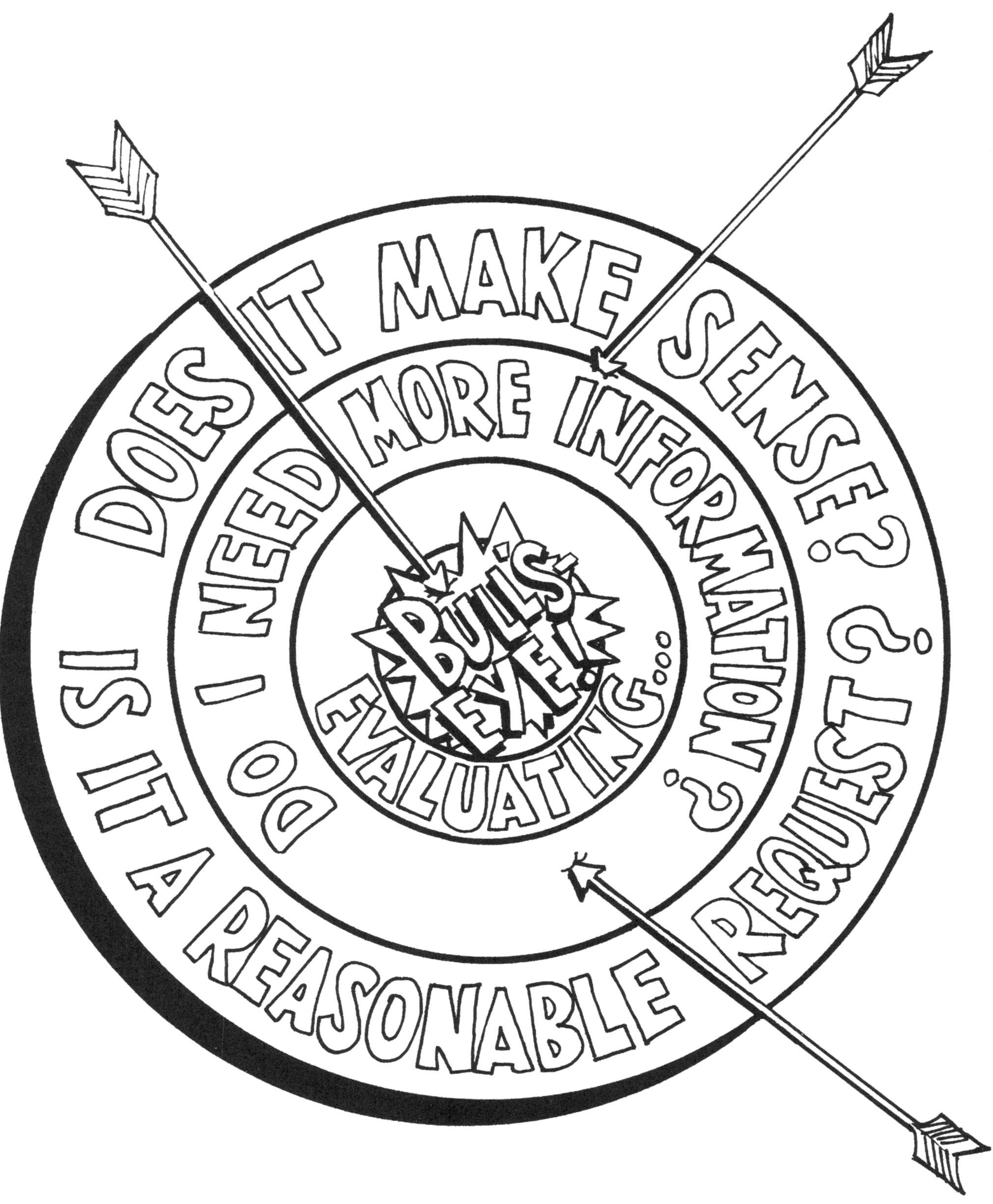
DOES IT MAKE SENSE?
I NEED MORE INFORMATION?
IS IT A REASONABLE REQUEST?
DO I NEED MORE INFORMATION?
EVALUATING...
BULL'S EYE!

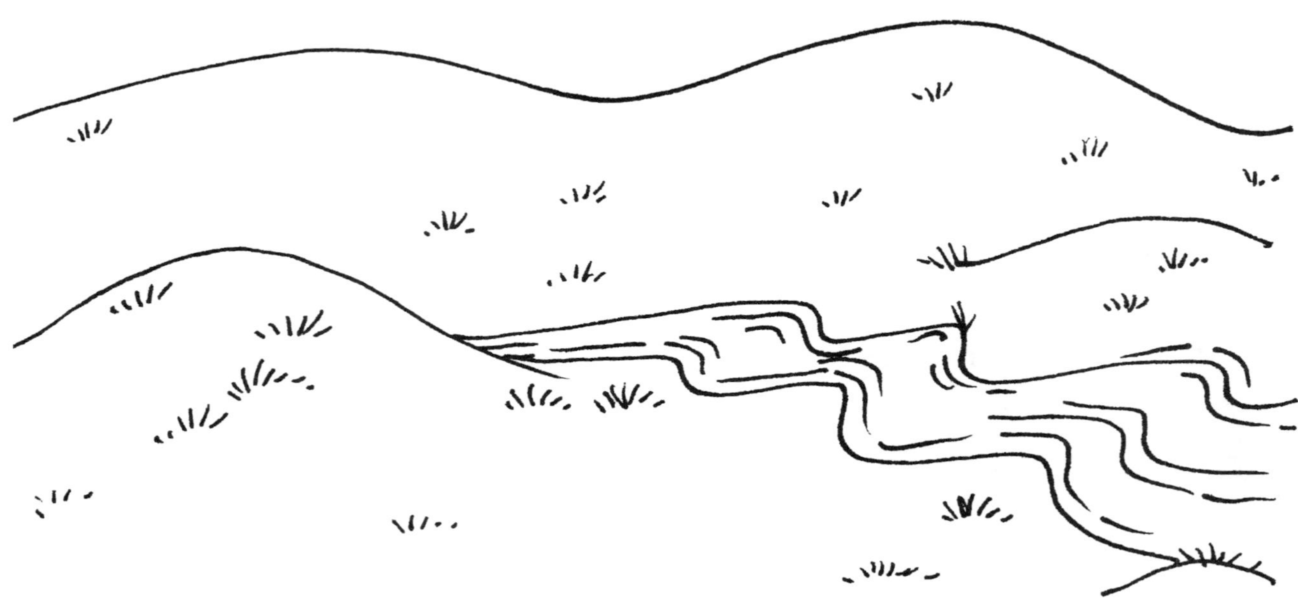

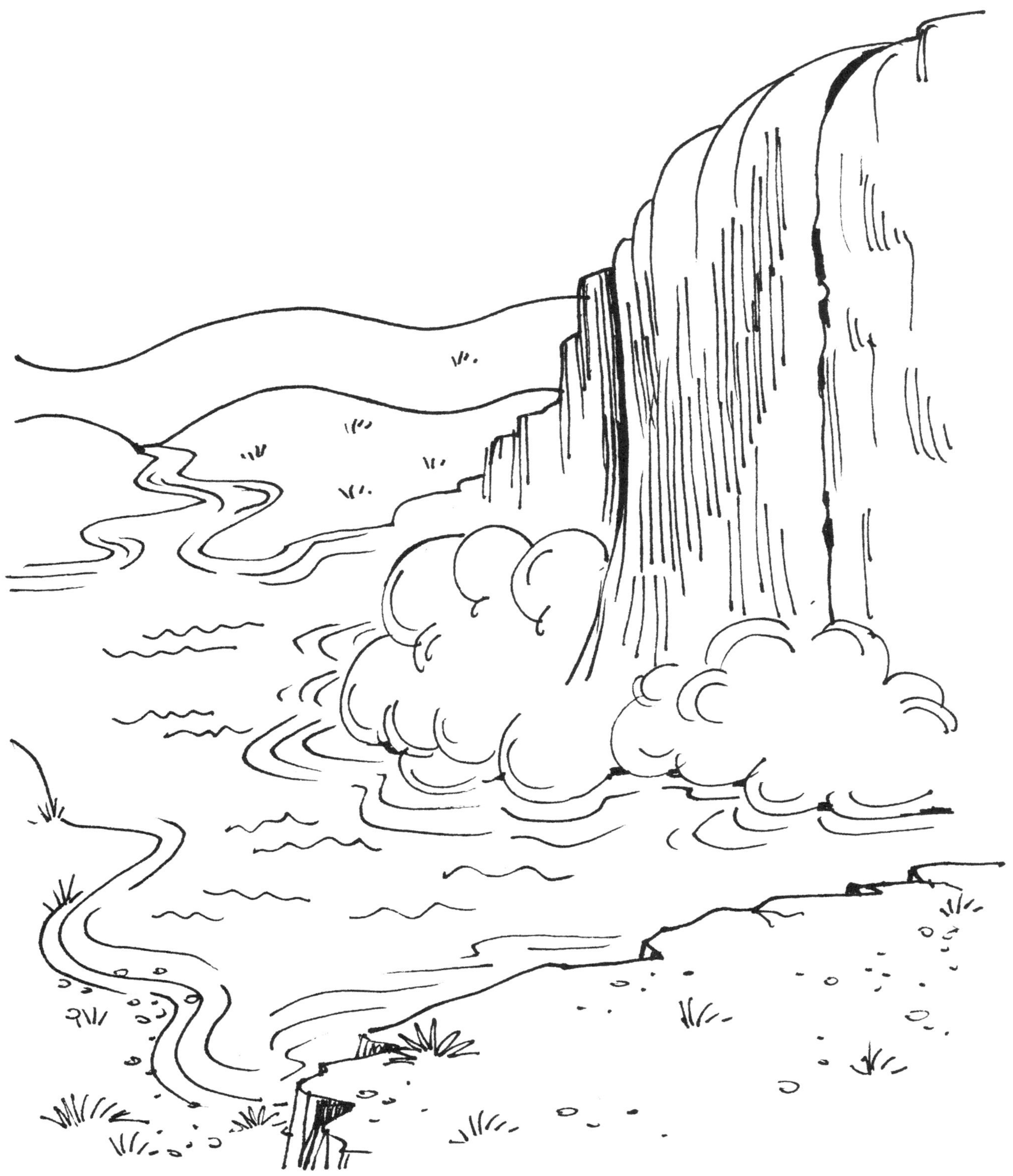

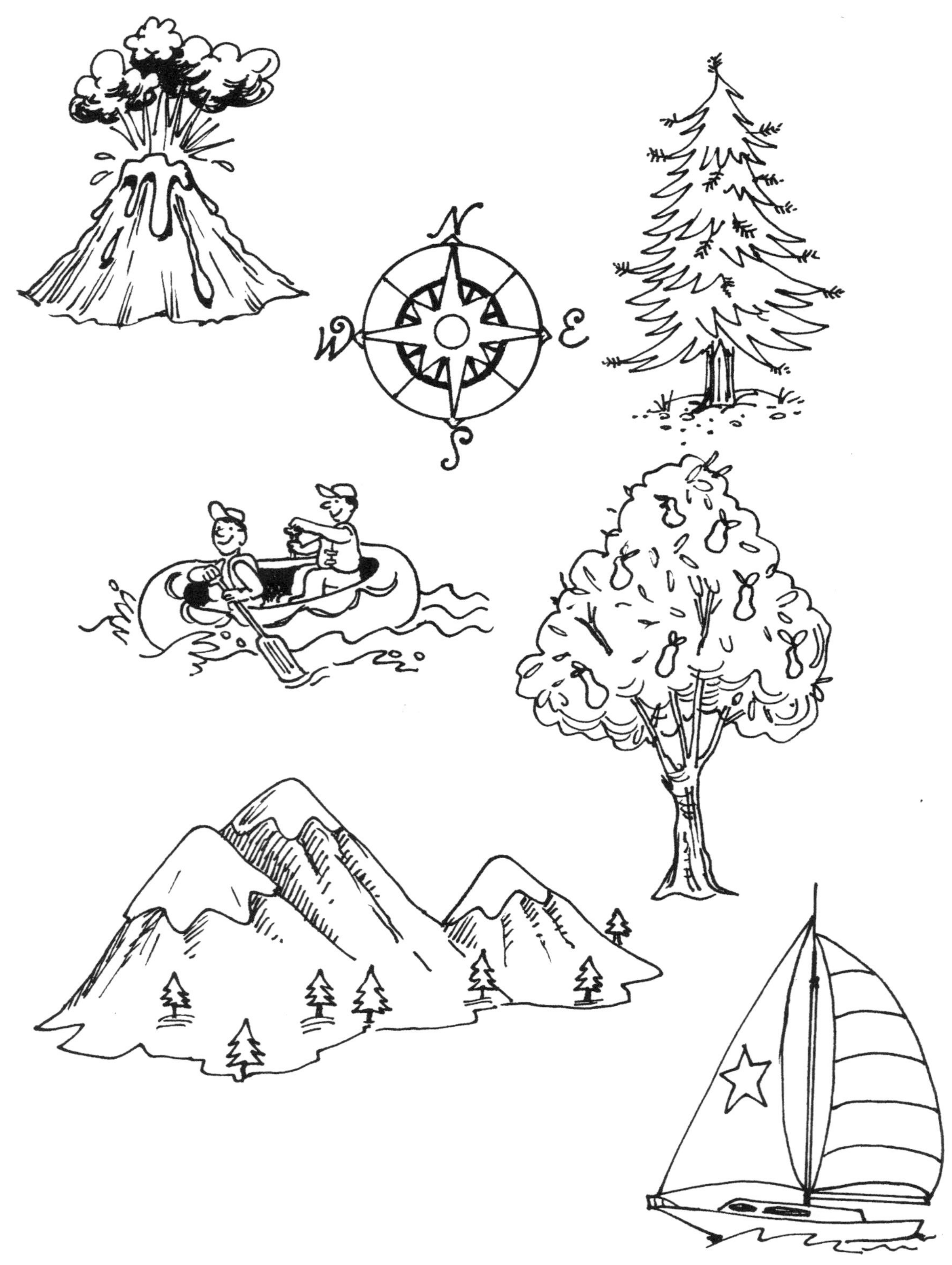
N
W
E
S

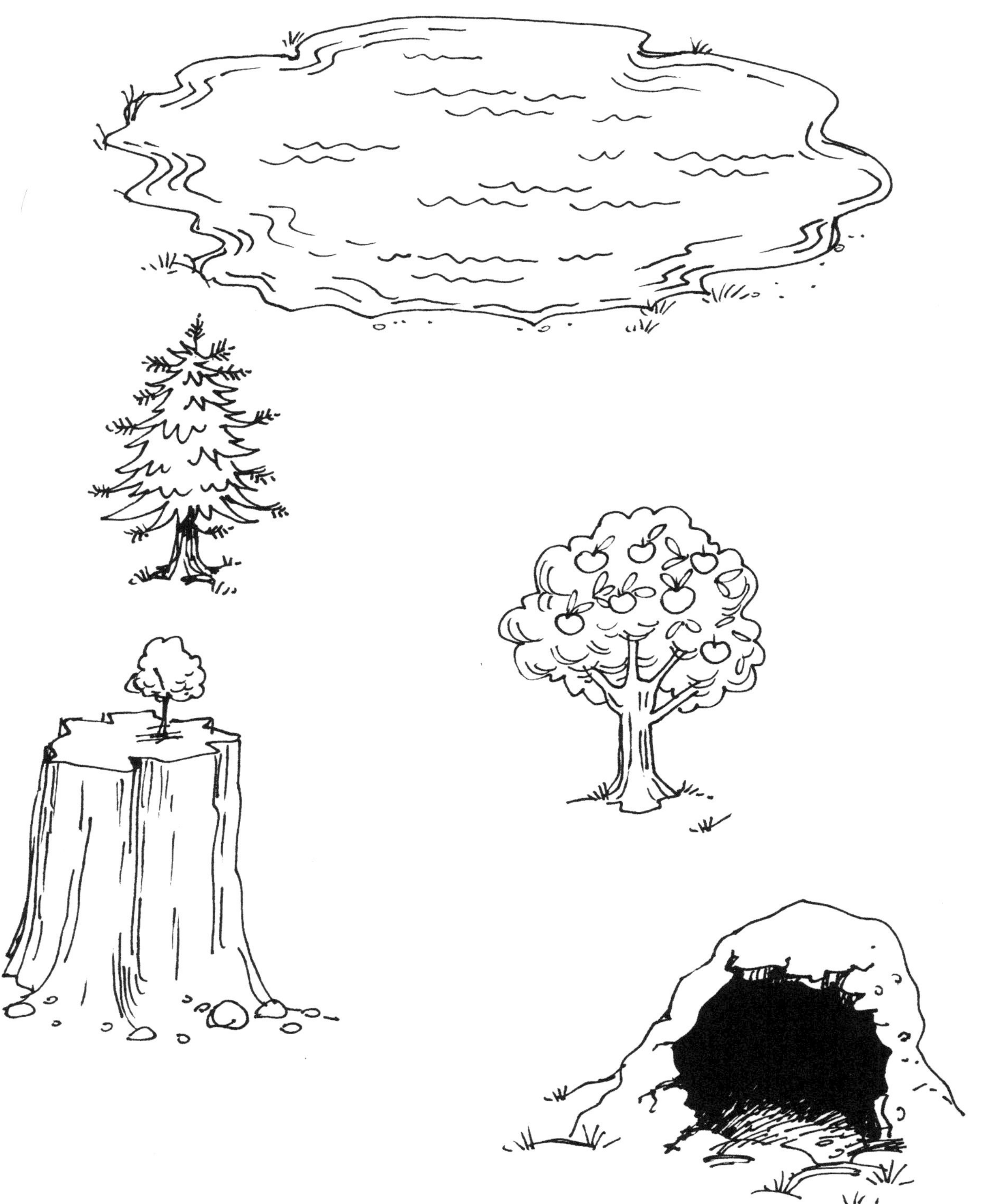

DETECT THE CLUES: FACT/OPINION (PART I)

GOAL

To improve evaluative listening

BACKGROUND INFORMATION

The main focus of the *Detect the Clues* strategy is to help students distinguish fact from opinion statements. This is an evaluative listening skill. The concepts stressed in the fact/opinion lesson will also be helpful in subsequent lessons or activities that involve the use of descriptive language. When describing, it is preferable to use specific, factual vocabulary such as, "The apple was crunchy and sweet," rather than to express an opinion such as, "The apple tasted good." This strategy is generally taught in two sessions so it is divided into Part I and Part II.

True understanding of fact/opinion does not develop until 10–12 years of age (Roeber, 1980), however, the purpose of this lesson is to help students begin to identify key words that signal opinions or statements of feelings. While identifying fact and opinion statements is an advanced thinking skill, students with a wide range of abilities can use the concrete cues provided by key words as a beginning step to distinguish fact from opinion.

OBJECTIVES

1. Use key words to identify fact and opinion statements from an advertisement.
2. Generate fact and opinion statements using key words.

MATERIALS

1. Chalkboard and chalk
2. *Detect the Clues* graphic (See page 64; duplicate and enlarge the graphic, color it, mount it onto poster board, and laminate it for durability, if desired.)
3. Two identical (except for color) maps (A state map is suggested, but any simple map will do. Mount one colorful map onto colorful construction paper and laminate it; mount the second map, but without color [i.e., black and white], onto manila construction paper, and laminate.)
4. Advertisements (Cut from magazines or newspapers)
5. *Crunch O's* advertisement (See page 65; duplicate one per student.)
6. Water-soluble markers (optional)

INTRODUCTION

Tie-in to Prior Learning

Review the skills learned in the last lesson regarding giving and receiving clear, precise directions, evaluating information, and requesting clarification when necessary. Explain that in this lesson students will be learning to listen to and evaluate information that is very tricky and requires expert evaluative listening.

Focus/Relevancy

1. Write the word *fact* on the board and ask what it means. Elicit the idea that information is real and can be demonstrated as real through proof. Say to the students,

   > *Today we are going to be detectives who detect clues to prove facts, but it may not be as easy as it sounds! Fact and opinion statements are used when telling what you know or feel about events or objects. A fact can be proven, for example, "I saw the best movie of the year this week. It received an Oscar for movie of the year."*

2. Write the word *opinion* on the board and ask what it means. Elicit the idea that an opinion is a belief that is not substantiated with proof. Present an example such as, "I saw the best movie ever this weekend. One of the characters was a talking pig."

3. Discuss the power of words and how easily they can influence us. Ask the students if they have ever been convinced to buy a product because of the advertisement, a friend's recommendation, or a commercial. Tell the students that they will be learning to recognize the key words that signal whether someone is telling a true fact or trying to convince them with their opinions.

LESSON ACTIVITIES

1. Hold up the two maps. Then hold up one map at a time and ask the students to tell which map they like better and why. If the students notice particular features on the colored map, point out the identical feature on the plain map. Discuss that people may prefer one map over the other, which is their opinion or their point of view. Note that the maps actually give identical information by saying,

   > *If we think one of these maps is better than the other, it would be based on our* personal preference *or* opinion *rather than any actual difference between the maps.* (Point to the word *opinion* written on the board.) *The information that each map represents is the same. The only difference depends on whether you like a map that is colorful rather than a plainer one.*

Expand on opinions. Have students generate several examples or provide examples students can relate to (e.g., not everyone thinks broccoli is a good-tasting food). Discuss the key words that might indicate a point of view, a preference, or an opinion and list them on the board. Ideas include: *think, like, feel* and sometimes words like *best, worst,* and *great.*

2. Explain that while the students may have preferred one map over the other, it is a fact that both of the maps give identical information. Ask someone to explain what a fact is. Use the maps to point out observable features (e.g., rivers, cities, highways, etc.). You can prove by looking at the map that the information is factual.

   Expand on facts. Discuss how certain statements can be proven to be factual just by observing (looking at, or experiencing) the information (e.g., "The Rollerblades are black, red, and green"). Facts can also be proven by looking in reference sources such as dictionaries, encyclopedias, or books. For thinking about facts and opinions at a higher level, have students consider how opinions could become facts (e.g., results of opinion polls). For the most part, facts will be true in all situations and can be agreed upon by all. Have students state various facts about their shoes, a favorite pet, toy, or sport.

3. Show the *Detect the Clues* poster. Explain the poster by saying,

   > *Our strategy is* Detect the Clues. *The poster shows Detective Dan looking for clues to separate facts from opinions. Let's read with whisper voices* (see page 13), *"A fact has a clue to prove it is true, but an opinion shows your point of view." Let's see if this strategy works.*

4. Show students the advertisements cut from magazines. Discuss statements made in advertisements that combine fact and opinion. Stress the idea that the advertisement is designed to influence you, the consumer (or buyer), to want or need the particular product. (Examples might include "Tony the Tiger says 'Frosted Flakes are GRRReat!,'" "If you wear Nike shoes, you will jump as high as Michael Jordan.")

5. Give each student a copy of the *Crunch-O's* advertisement. Read the advertisement for Crunch-O's together. Explain that the students' job will be to underline the statements of fact and circle statements showing opinions. Check for understanding. Divide students into pairs and have students work with their partners to complete the activity together. (The page could be laminated and used again if students use water-soluble markers.)

6. Have pairs share their findings (i.e., the statements of fact and opinion that they found). Help the students determine if the one fact statement could be proved (i.e., the nutritional information

on the box would help to determine if there are eight vitamins and iron). Ask a student pair to share the opinion statements found and have them identify the key words. Students quickly discover the key words that show feelings or opinions.

CLOSURE

Summarize the lesson, review its relevance to students, and tie it to future learning. Encourage students to continue to be fact/opinion detectives and to listen for those key words that let them know whether a statement is a fact that can be proven or whether it is strictly someone's point of view.

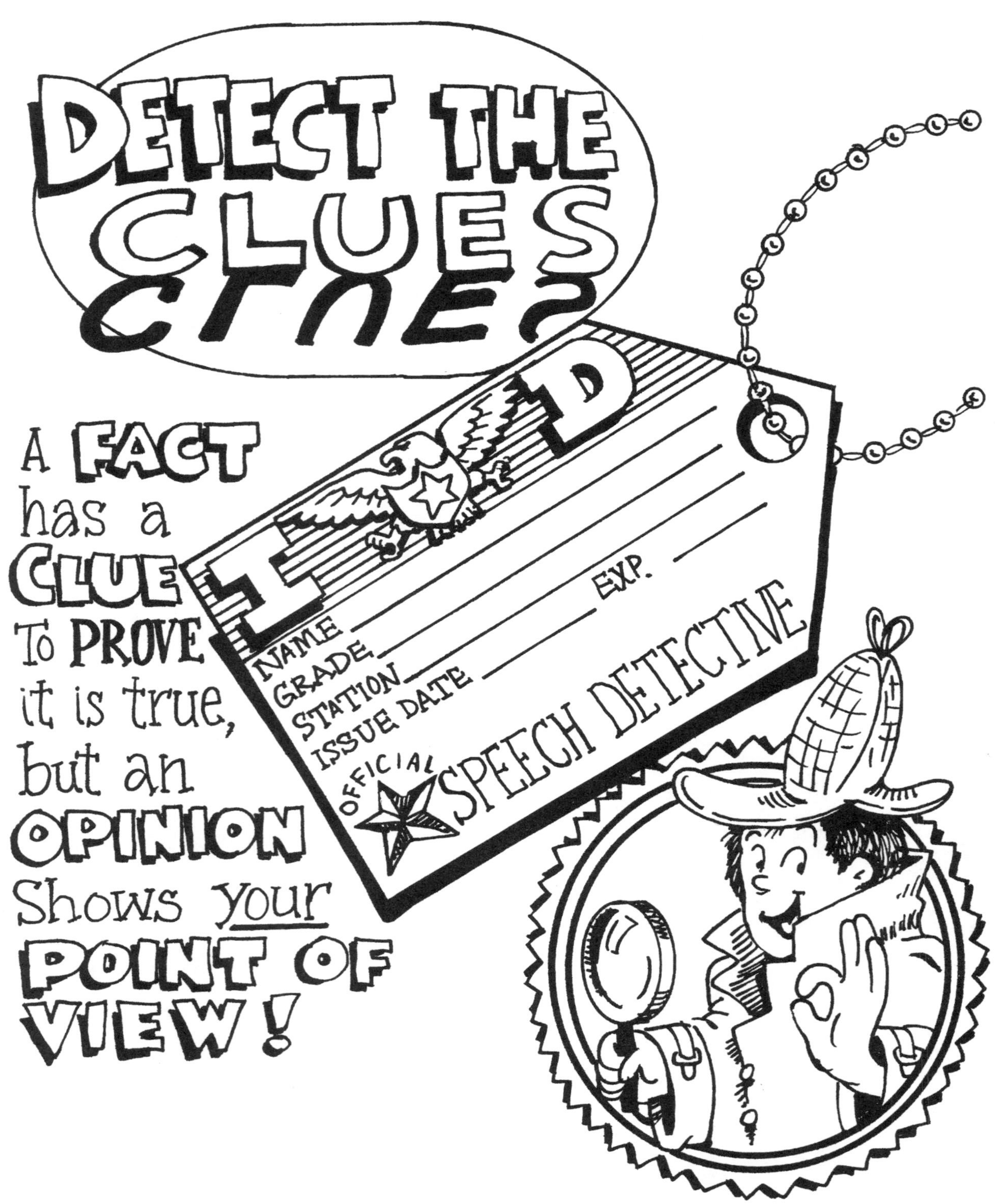
DETECT THE CLUES
A FACT has a CLUE To PROVE it is true, but an OPINION Shows your POINT OF VIEW!
I D
NAME
GRADE
STATION
ISSUE DATE
EXP.
OFFICIAL SPEECH DETECTIVE

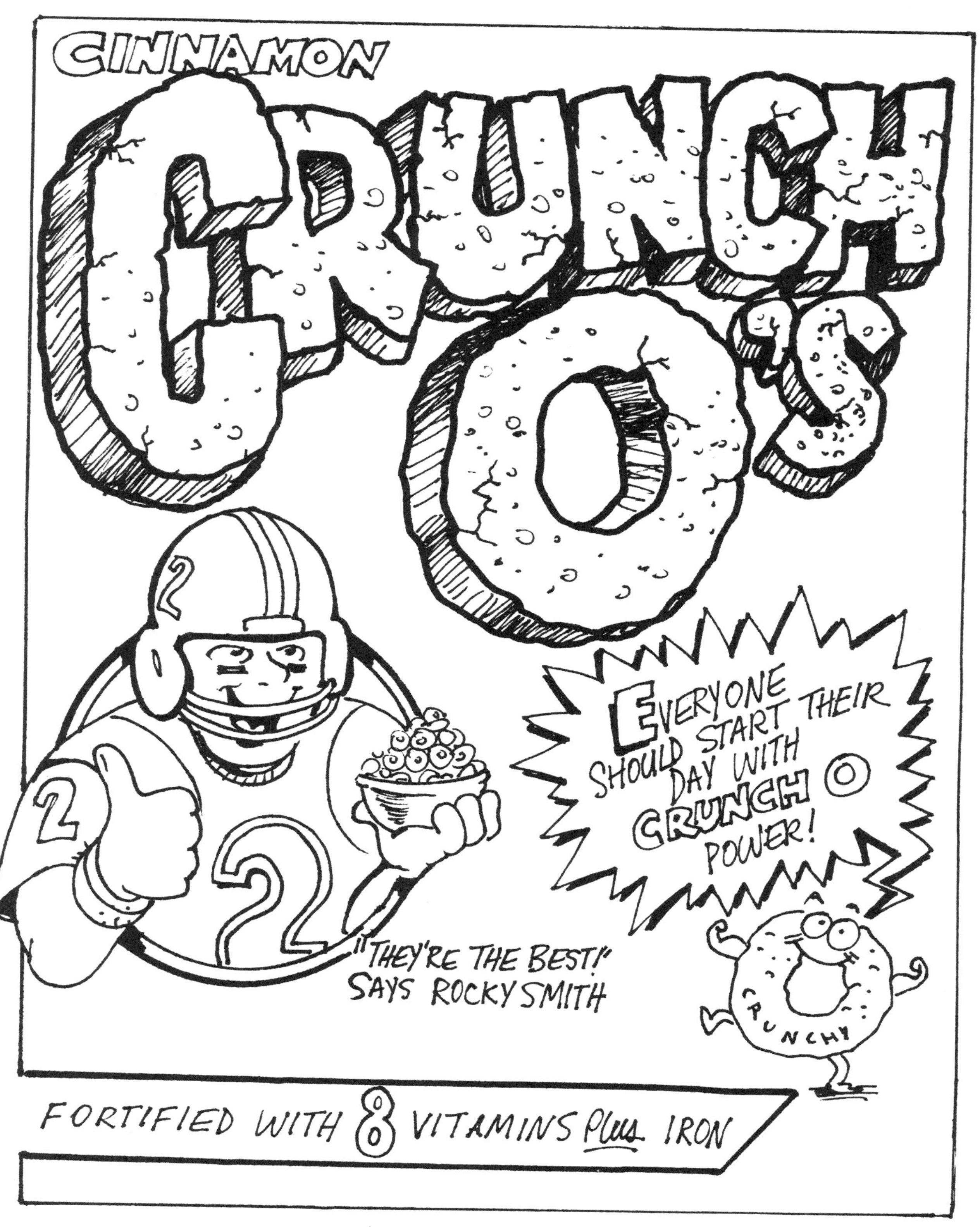
CINNAMON
CRUNCH O'S
EVERYONE SHOULD START THEIR DAY WITH CRUNCH O POWER!
"THEY'RE THE BEST!" SAYS ROCKY SMITH
CRUNCHY
FORTIFIED WITH 8 VITAMINS Plus IRON

DETECT THE CLUES: FACT/OPINION (PART II)

GOAL

To improve comprehension skill

BACKGROUND INFORMATION

The main focus of the *Detect the Clues* strategy is to help students distinguish fact from opinion statements. The concepts stressed in the fact/opinion lesson will also be helpful in subsequent lessons or activities that involve the use of descriptive language. When describing, it is preferable to use specific, factual vocabulary such as, "The apple was crunchy and sweet," rather than to express an opinion such as, "The apple tasted good."

True understanding of fact/opinion does not develop until 10–12 years of age (Roeber, 1980), however, the purpose of this lesson is to help students begin to identify key words that signal opinions or statements of feelings. While identifying fact and opinion statements is an advanced thinking skill, students with a wide range of abilities can use the concrete cues provided by key words as a beginning step to distinguish fact from opinion.

OBJECTIVES

1. Generate fact and opinion statements.
2. Write an advertisement using fact and opinion statements.

MATERIALS

1. *Detect the Clues* graphic (Created earlier)
2. *Little Sister for Sale* (1992) by Morse Hamilton and Giogia Fiammenghi (optional)
3. Advertisements cut from magazines or newspapers
4. Old magazines or newspapers for cutting out advertisements
5. Glue or glue stick (One per pair of students)
6. Scissors (One per pair of students)
7. *Advertisement* (See page 68; duplicate one per pair of students.)

INTRODUCTION

Tie-in to Prior Learning

Review the *Detect the Clues* strategy using the poster. Have students recall fact and opinion statements that are used in advertisements or commercials. Review key words that help to identify opinions.

Focus/Relevancy

Show the advertisements cut from newspapers or magazines. Highlight how advertisements are sometimes pieced together to form an entire page and that ad space is expensive. Designers of ads want to write statements that will influence buyers. In this activity, students will be ad designers.

LESSON ACTIVITIES

1. As an option, read the story *Little Sister for Sale.* Summarize the story by discussing a sample advertisement for the "little sister." Identify the characters who are the buyer-consumer, seller-advertiser, and what the product is. Model writing an advertisement using two statements of fact and two opinion statements regarding the little sister. Point out how the use of illustrations or pictures makes an ad more interesting.

2. Pair students. Distribute the newspapers, magazines, glue, and scissors to each pair of students. Also distribute the *Advertisement* activity page. Have students cut out a product from the magazine or newspaper that they like and glue it to their activity sheets. Tell the students to imagine that they have a wonderful product to sell and they must create the advertisement to fill the page. Relate this activity to commercials on television. Ask the students what makes them want to buy a product based on TV commercials. Remind students of the words used in advertisements such as *best, unbelievable,* and *zippy*.

3. Explain to students that they will be the ad writers today. They must include two factual statements and two opinion statements. (If students have difficulty with this activity, using concrete objects [e.g., a plastic, glow-in-the-dark snake, a stuffed bunny, or a rubber ball] sometimes helps to generate ideas.) Have each pair create their ads. Allow students time to be creative. Although some student pairs will be quite independent, others will need guidance in selecting their product and getting started. Allow each pair time to share their advertisements with the large group.

CLOSURE

Summarize the lesson, review its relevance to students, and tie it to future learning. Encourage the students to continue to be fact/opinion detectives and to listen for those key words that let them know whether a statement is a fact that can be proven or whether it is strictly someone's point of view.

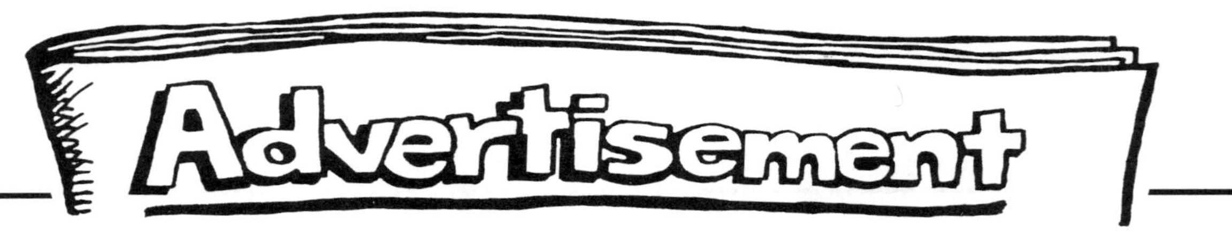

Names: ______________________________ Date: ________________

HIT THE BULL'S-EYE and DETECT THE CLUES FOLLOW-UP ACTIVITIES

GOAL

To reinforce and review *Hit the Bull's-Eye* and *Detect the Clues* strategies

BACKGROUND INFORMATION

The main focus of this lesson is to review the previous two strategies. The strategy guide review pages will be compiled with similar pages into a booklet at the end of the school year. This booklet, along with a vacation calendar, provide a means of practicing with family members and reinforcing skills throughout a school break. Although some educators may choose to do the strategy guide pages and homework activities at the end of each lesson, others prefer delayed reinforcement to strengthen knowledge of strategies, concepts, and vocabulary covered within the lessons. Using a small representation of the strategy poster, the strategy guide pages include the specific vocabulary from the lessons. An application component is provided on the second pages of the strategy guides. Students may do reflective writing about how the strategy is or can be useful to them.

OBJECTIVES

1. Tell and write the major components of the *Hit the Bull's-Eye* and *Detect the Clues* strategies.
2. Reflect and write about how the strategies will help at home, at school, and in the community.
3. Share strategy information with family members and complete the application activities.

MATERIALS

1. *Hit the Bull's-Eye* poster (Created earlier)
2. *Detect the Clues* poster (Created earlier)
3. *Hit the Bull's-Eye Strategy Guide* (See pages 71–72; duplicate one per student.)
4. *Detect the Clues Strategy Guide* (See pages 73–74; duplicate one per student.)
5. *Hit the Bull's-Eye Homework Activity* (See page 75; duplicate one per student.)
6. *Detect the Clues Homework Activity* (See page 76; duplicate one per student.)

INTRODUCTION

Tie-in to Prior Learning

Refer students to the initial goal-setting activity (see pages 19–20) and their completed goal sheets. Discuss that when setting their listening goals, they talked about some of the times and/or places that presented problems with listening effectively. Point out that they have learned two more strategies that will help them improve and move toward achieving their goals. Display the posters and review the *Hit the Bull's-Eye* and *Detect the Clues* strategies.

Focus/Relevancy

Review the importance of the *Strategy Guide Booklet* which will be a collection of the student's guide pages for each strategy learned. The booklet will help them become better communicators by helping them remember all the strategies they will be learning. Explain to students that new pages will be added as new strategies are learned and remind them that the booklet of strategies will be theirs to keep.

LESSON ACTIVITIES

1. Distribute the *Hit the Bull's-Eye Strategy Guid*e pages and the *Detect the Clues Strategy Guide* pages and have students complete them. Students should demonstrate they know the strategies by completing the blank lines. Point out to students the choices are included on the page. Refer to the graphics and have them displayed for the students.

2. On the second page of each strategy guide, have students write how each particular strategy has helped them or will help them at school, at home, or in the community. Brainstorm ideas (e.g., "When I don't understand the teacher's directions in math class, I will ask for clarification," "I gave clear directions to my friend to get to my house," "I recognize the words that show opinions rather than the facts").

3. Hand out the *Hit the Bull's-Eye* and the *Detect the Clues Homework Activity* pages and discuss them. Reinforce the importance of sharing this information with family members, and the ease and fun of doing these assignments. They will only take a few minutes to complete, but students can impress their family with what they have learned! Have a reward system established to encourage students to bring their homework activity pages back to school signed by a family member.

CLOSURE

Summarize the lesson, review its relevance to students, and tie it to future learning. Discuss the objectives that were completed in this review (i.e., the students can tell and write the *Hit the Bull's-Eye* and *Detect the Clues* strategies; they can tell how they will use the strategies; they know the strategies well enough to share them with their family members).

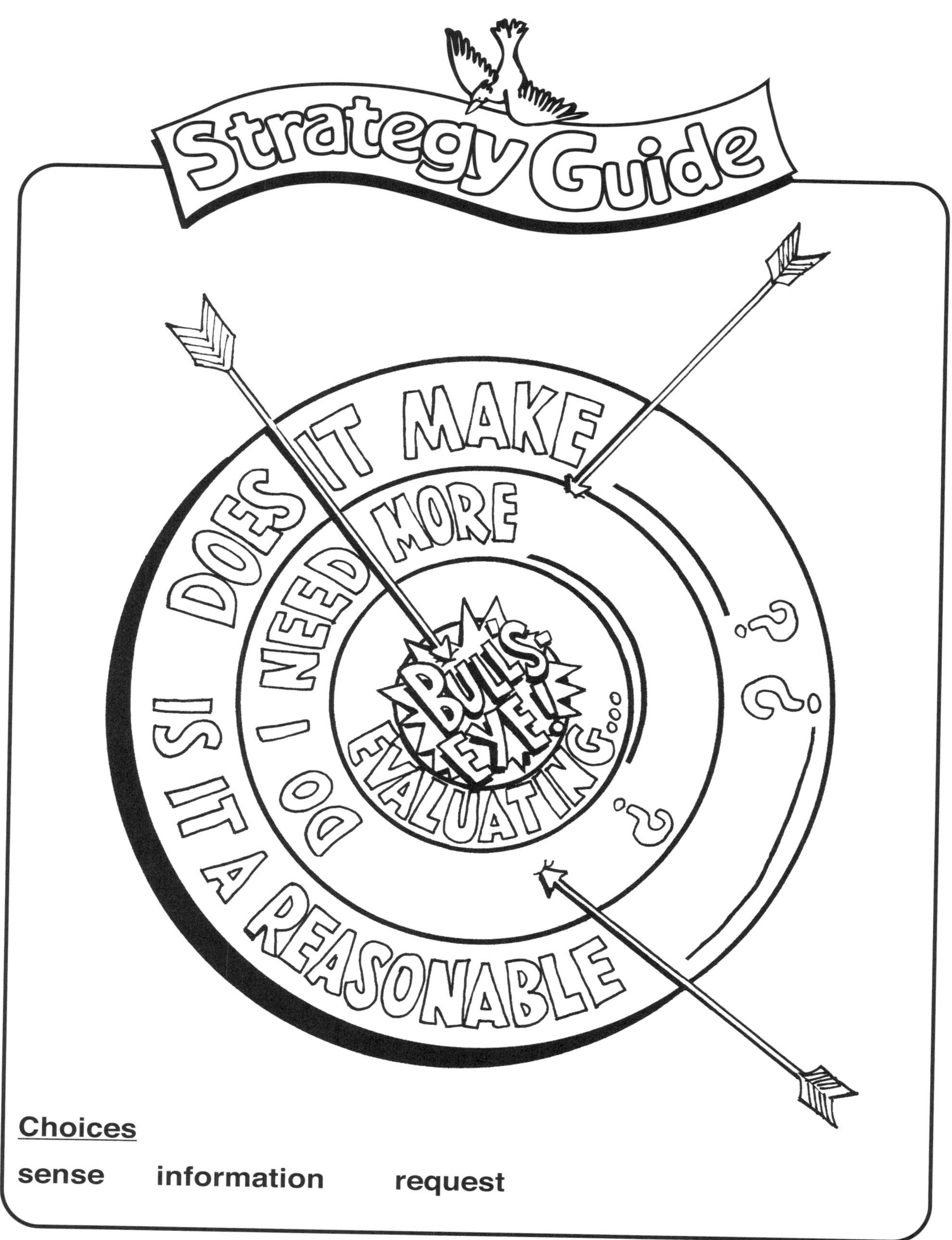

Choices

sense information request

Hit the Bull's-Eye: Giving and Receiving Directions

Name: ______________________________ Date: ______________

Directions: Write a sentence about how you have used or will use the strategy in each place.

At home, I ____

____

____

____

____

____

At school, I ____

____

____

____

____

____

In my community, I ____

____

____

____

____

____

Strategy Guide
DETECT THE CLUES
A FACT
has a
CLUE To
it is true,
but an
OPINION
Shows your
NAME
GRADE
STATION
ISSUE DATE
EXP.
OFFICIAL
SPEECH DETECTIVE

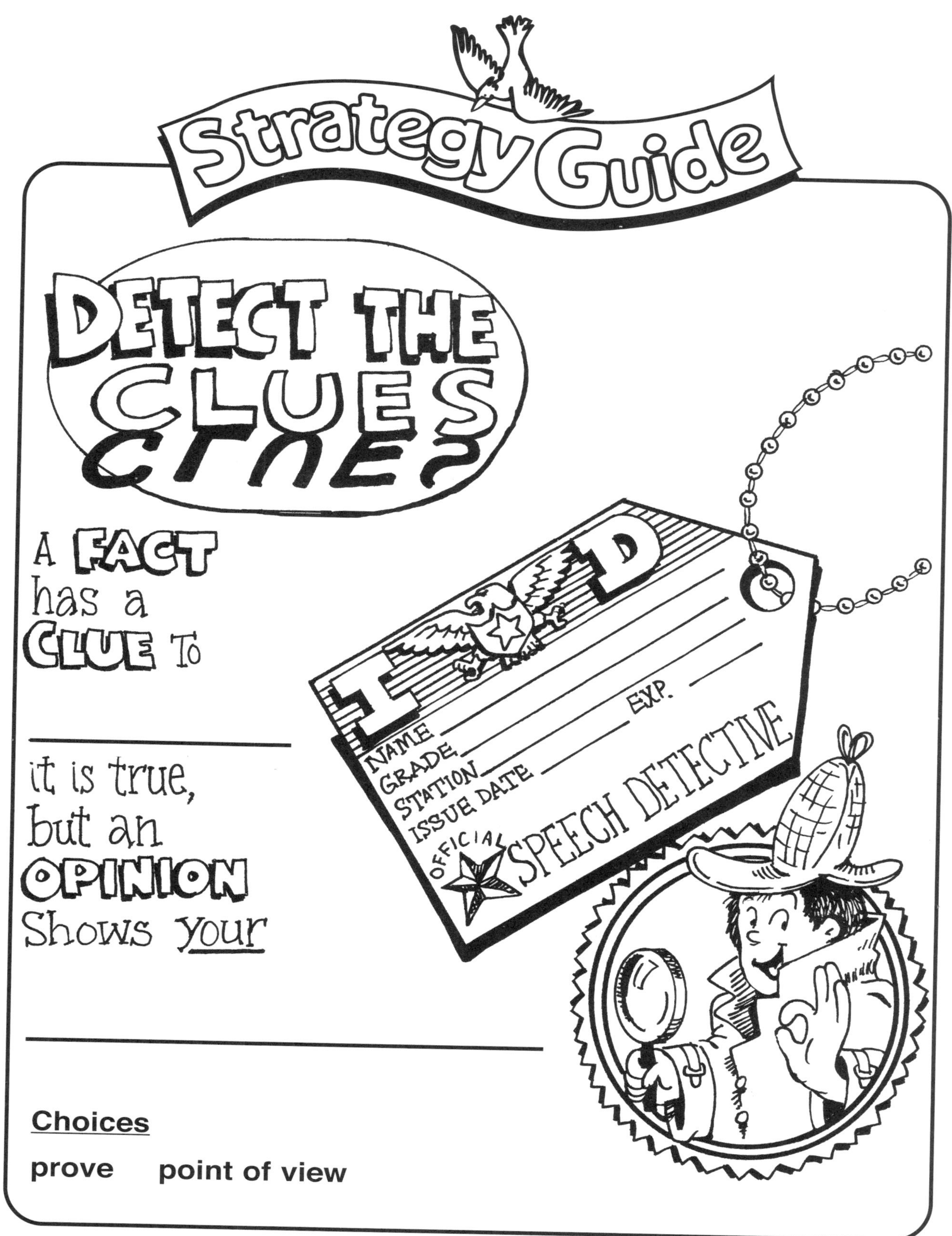

Choices

prove **point of view**

Detect the Clues: Fact/Opinion

Name: ______________________________ Date: ____________

Directions: Write a sentence about how you have used or will use the strategy in each place.

At home, I ______________________________

____

____

____

____

____

At school, I ______________________________

____

____

____

____

____

In my community, I ______________________________

____

____

____

____

____

Homework Activity

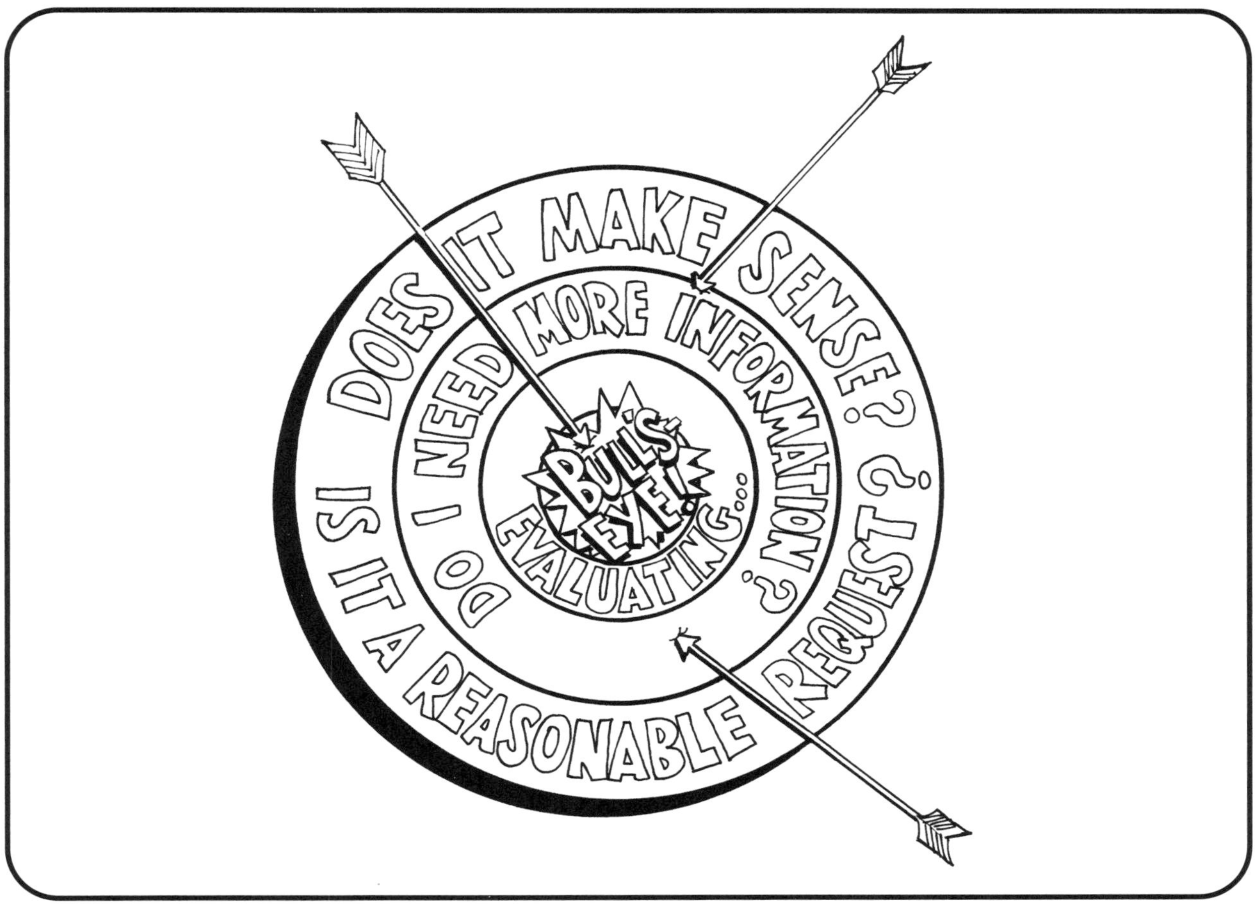

Dear Family,

1. Have your child explain the *Hit the Bull's-Eye* strategy and tell why it's important to be specific when you give or follow directions.
2. Ask your child to give directions for finding something in his or her bedroom. Encourage your child to be specific.
3. Have your child give detailed directions for making his or her favorite snack.
4. Ask your child to explain what it means to *ask for clarification.* Have him or her demonstrate the "polite" way to ask. (Hint: "Excuse me, but did you mean…").
5. If your child completes these activities, please sign below and return this form to school.

Family Member: ________________________________ Date: ________________

Homework Activity

DETECT THE CLUES
CLUES
A FACT has a CLUE To PROVE it is true, but an OPINION Shows your POINT OF VIEW!
ID
NAME
GRADE
STATION
ISSUE DATE
EXP.
OFFICIAL SPEECH DETECTIVE

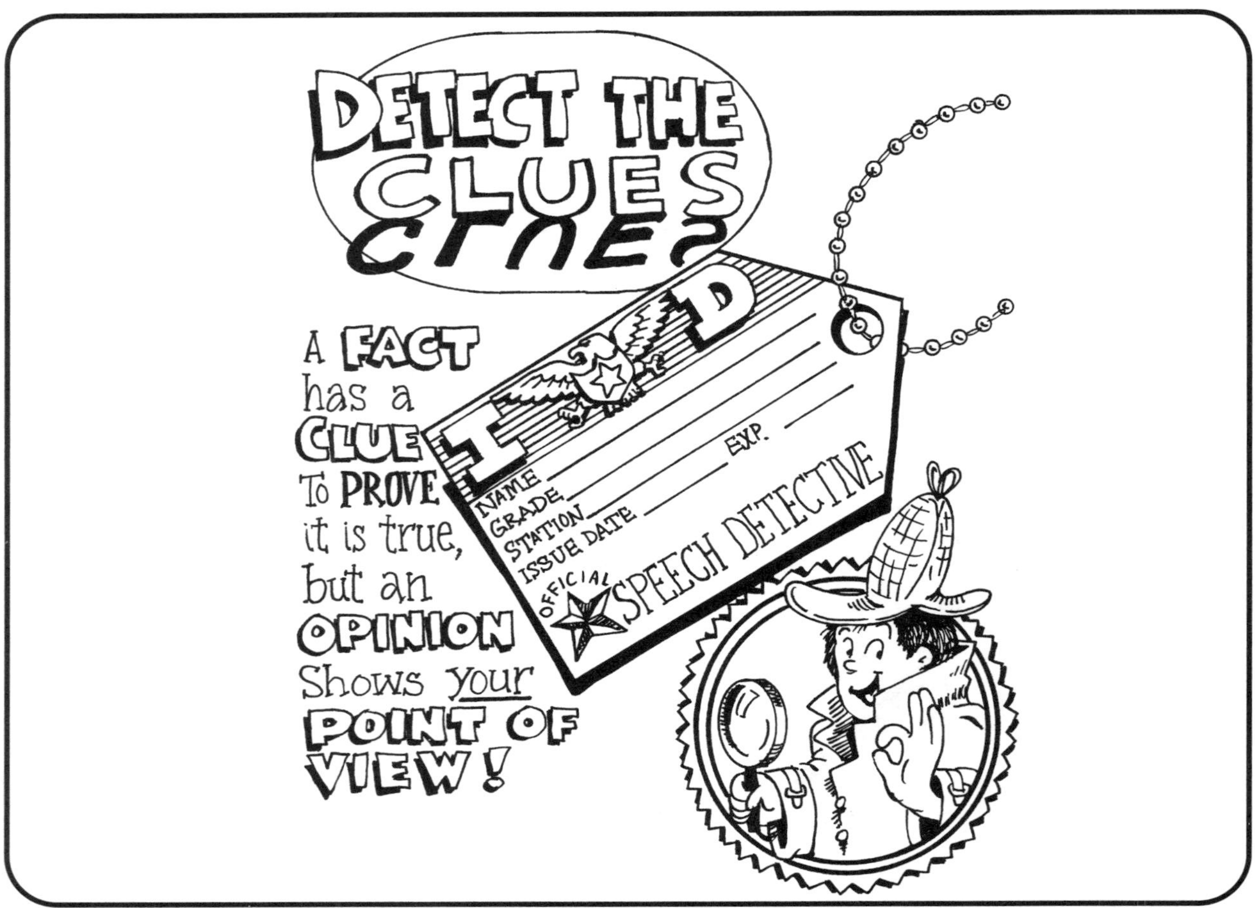

Dear Family,

1. Have your child explain the *Detect the Clues* strategy and tell why it's important to know a fact from an opinion.
2. Have your child tell you three key words that signal an opinion statement.
3. Ask your child to give a fact and an opinion statement about a vegetable.
4. Ask your child to give a fact and opinion statement about a snack food.
5. Tell your child two facts and two opinions you have about a movie you've seen.
6. If your child completes these activities, please sign below and return this form to school.

Family Member: ________________________________ Date: ________________

UNIT TWO

GOAL SETTING ACTIVITY TWO

GOAL

To encourage self-improvement through goal setting

BACKGROUND INFORMATION

The main focus of this lesson is to help students learn the steps for goal setting (i.e., identifying a need, formulating a goal, practicing the steps to reach the goal, revising a goal as needed, and evaluating progress toward meeting a goal). Rather than expecting students to set goals independently, the goal-setting process is modeled. The communication goal could be directed by you, but the reflection on how the goal might be useful will be individual for each student, since each student's use of the skills will be different. A few example goals for this unit are:

1. Improve describing skills;
2. Use interesting words in descriptions;
3. Use specific vocabulary when telling about categories; and
4. Improve categorization skills.

OBJECTIVES

1. Understand the following goal-setting concepts: achieving a goal, revising a goal, and evaluating progress made.
2. Evaluate progress on achieving previously set goals.
3. Tell how previous goals were met.
4. Write a new goal.

MATERIALS

1. *My Goals #2* (See page 82; duplicate one per student.)
2. *My Goals #1* (Completed in *Goal Setting Activity One*)
3. Chalkboard and chalk

INTRODUCTION

Tie-in to Prior Learning

Remind students that in *Goal Setting Activity One,* they had identified specific areas of listening which could be focused on for improvement. Review the terms *goal, achieve,* and *skills.* Refer to the initial goal-setting activity in which the students discussed the idea that achieving a goal takes practice. Review the strategies that the students have been learning and practicing in the previous lessons.

Focus/Relevancy

1. Stress that learning is easier when goals are set and there is a plan for practicing. Remind students that setting goals can help them achieve or accomplish many different skills both in school, at home, and someday at a job.

2. Say to the students,

   It is time to evaluate how we did on our previous goals and then set new ones. When we evaluate our work, we are deciding if we have done our best work or a good job. Soccer players who need to work on their skills could evaluate progress on a kicking goal by seeing if the ball kicked landed where they wanted it. If the ball is too far to the side, or not high enough, they need to continue practicing that skill. We can evaluate our progress on listening skills by deciding how we have used our skills at school, at home, and in the community.

LESSON ACTIVITIES

1. Give each student a copy of *My Goals #2* and their completed *My Goals #1.* Write the words *achieve, revise,* and *repeat* on the board. Explain the meaning of the words. Model using self-evaluation (e.g., "I went to a meeting that was really long. I listened carefully for important information and requested clarification when I did not hear or understand. After a while, I really had to make an effort not to draw on my note pad or flip through my materials!") to evaluate goals set during *Goal Setting Activity One*. Have students check whether they achieved their goals or whether they need to revise their goals. Before marking their goal sheets, encourage students to reflect on ways they practiced their steps to reach their goals.

2. Remind students that, just as a soccer player needs to concentrate and practice skills needing improvement, once the goal is achieved, they will need to continue to practice and repeat the skill while targeting another skill area for improvement.

3. Point out the "My new goal is" sentence on the goal sheet. The next two skills targeted are describing and categorization. Discuss the value of improving these two areas by saying,

   We have learned a lot about listening and now we are ready to use these skills to help us learn about being better speakers and writers. Describing is an important school skill and if you aren't very comfortable with thinking about what that is, we'll need to set describing as a goal. Have you ever had to use describing words or write a descriptive paragraph? Was it hard? How many of you could use some tools to make it easier to think of describing words?

Write a goal such as *Improve describing skills* on the board. Repeat the process with *categorization.* Tell students that they cannot get through a day without doing some kind of categorizing or "grouping." Refer to how clothes are categorized in a closet, how laundry is grouped before washing, or animals are grouped in science, etc. Write a goal such as *Improve categorization skills* on the board for the students to add to their goal sheet.

CLOSURE

Summarize the lesson, repeat its relevance to students, and tie it to future learning. Discuss that the students have set important goals and next time will begin working on the first skill to achieve their describing goal. Remind the students that by signing and dating the top line they are promising to concentrate and work on their goal. The second line is for a family member to sign. Students can teach their families about describing and categorizing as these skills are learned. Offer a tangible or social reward for returning the goal sheet if desired.

My Goals #2

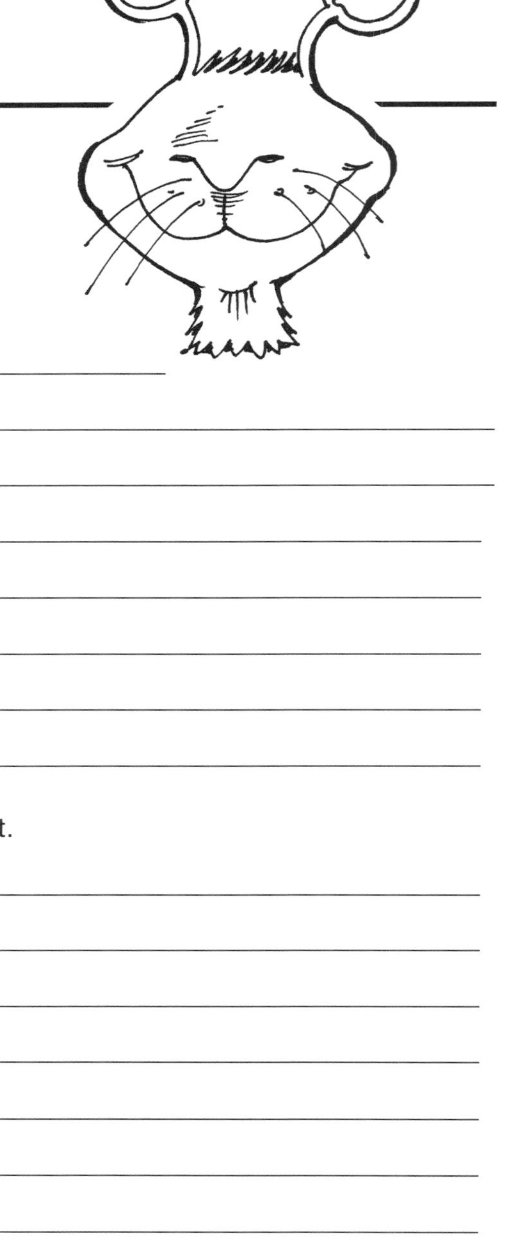

In the last unit, my goals were: ____________________

____

Now, at home, I ______________________________

____

Now, at school, I ______________________________

____

Now, in the community, I ______________________________

____

☐ I achieved my goal, but will keep practicing it.

☐ I need to revise my goal by ______________________________

____

My new goal is ______________________________

____

At home, I will ______________________________

____

At school, I will ______________________________

____

In the community, I will ______________________________

____

Name: ____________________ Date: __________

Teacher: ____________________ Date: __________

Family Member: ____________________ Date: __________

CREATURE CREATOR: DESCRIBING USING VISION

GOAL

To use precise descriptors in expressive language

BACKGROUND INFORMATION

The *Creature Creator* lesson begins a series of lessons that work to build vocabulary knowledge and flexibility in word use. The main focus of the *Creature Creator* strategy is to help students use size, shape, color, and distinctive feature characteristics when describing items seen. Visual information is specifically highlighted in this lesson. Other senses are addressed in the next lesson, *It Makes Sense*. Many academic tasks require students to describe visually without the benefit of using all of their senses, as in an assignment or activity requiring students to describe strictly from a picture. In this lesson, students are encouraged to use attributes that are visually observable although the attribute might also fit another sense (e.g., a fuzzy attribute can be seen and felt).

OBJECTIVES

1. Use size, shape, color, and distinctive features when describing characteristics of an object seen.
2. Write a descriptive sentence using size, shape, color, and distinctive features.

MATERIALS

1. *Creature Creator* graphic (See page 87; duplicate and enlarge the graphic, color it, mount it onto poster board, and laminate it for durability, if desired.)
2. Two food items (One that is desirable to eat [e.g., a small Tootsie Roll] and another that is undesirable to eat [e.g., an old, unscraped carrot])
3. *Weird Creature Parts* (See page 88–92; duplicate onto heavy stock paper, cut apart, and color; make at least one of each body part for each student.)
4. *Visual Description* (See page 93; duplicate one per student and one per pair of students.)
5. Objects to describe (See step 4.)

INTRODUCTION

Tie-in to Prior Learning

Remind students that in the *Detect the Clues* strategy they talked about listening carefully for key words that signaled fact and opinion statements and used the key words to write advertisements. Explain that in this lesson they will be using factual words to describe what they see in a clear, precise way also.

Focus/Relevancy

1. Say to the students,

   We are going to practice being scientists or investigators by using our observational skills. Why would these occupations require you to be a good observer? (Give students time to respond.) *What senses might you use when observing?* (Give students time to respond.) *I brought some special items with me today.* (Hold up the disgusting looking carrot and the Tootsie Roll.) *I'm going to let you request one of these items as a treat for later. Who can tell me what the word* request *means?* (Discuss appropriate ways to make requests.) *I have one special rule before we begin; you must request the item by describing what you see; you may not request the item by its name. Does anyone need clarification of the instructions?*

2. Without modeling, have students request a treat. They should want the desirable treat (e.g., the Tootsie Roll) over the undesirable one (e.g., the carrot) and attempt to describe the desirable treat visually (e.g., "Could I have the brown treat?"). When a child asks using a visual characteristic, give them the treat. Tell students they must set the treat down on the corner of their desks until you give them permission to eat it. As the students begin to understand how to use descriptive words to make their requests clear, discuss the characteristics they're naming (i.e., color, size, shape, or a distinctive feature).

   HINT
   The term d*istinctive feature* may require more clarification and examples. (Use the golf clap [see page 13] to clap out the syllables in the word *distinctive.*) Discuss what makes something different or unusual from the things around it. An example might be when someone comes to your classroom and doesn't know a student's name, they describe the student by hair color, clothing, or something that makes them unique from the other students around them.

   Also, students need to realize that size is a relative term and depends on the size of the other items to which one item is compared (e.g., a mouse is big when compared to an ant, small when compared to an elephant, and medium-sized in relation to both). Give students a referent point when asking them to describe the size of an object.

   If students name a characteristic that does not use vision (e.g., "Could I have the sweet treat?") affirm what they're describing, but ask for characteristics that can be seen. After all visual characteristics have been named and discussed, let those who have not had an opportunity to earn their treat, review the characteristics as a group. Students may eat their treats at your discretion.

3. Discuss how successful description of visual characteristics resulted in each student receiving the treat requested. Relate this experience to other situations such as asking someone to buy a particular item for school. If a student does not describe exactly what is needed, the wrong item might be purchased.

LESSON ACTIVITIES

1. Show the *Creature Creator* poster. Demonstrate how certain characteristics could be fed into the machine to make a Tootsie Roll. A cylinder shape, a small size, a brown color, a wrapper of white, brown, and red, could be fed into the machine and might come out as a Tootsie Roll. By using these characteristics, students can help others picture exactly what they are describing.

2. Tell students they are going to practice using specific words to describe objects. Give each student either a head, a body, or a feet picture from the *Weird Creature Parts* and a *Visual Description* activity page. Tell students to use the *Visual Description* activity page to organize their thoughts into a clear description that includes size, shape, color, and distinctive features of the creature part. When the students have finished documenting their observations, gather all the creature parts and line them up on a chalk tray or a bulletin board where students can see them. Have each student read their creature part description and have another student find the part that matches the description (e.g., "Find the head that is oval, purple, and has a green tongue sticking out"). To make this lesson more challenging, give each student three parts (i.e., a head, a body, and feet) of a creature to describe and then have other students guess which pictures fit the description. Also color the parts so there is more than one part of the same color (e.g., two feet have purple shoes, three bodies are green). This helps students focus on distinctive features and requires more precise descriptions.

   Take advantage of opportunities when communication problems occur and when clarification is needed. Discuss why the breakdown occurred, whether it was the speaker's or the listener's fault, and how it could be corrected.

3. Model combining ideas in sentence form. Describe one particular part or describe the entire creature. Talk about combining two ideas with the conjunctions *and* or *but* (e.g., "Find the head that is oval, purple, and has a green tongue sticking out," "Find the feet that are __ but not ___"). Help students write and then share their sentences with the large group. Do this as a group for younger students.

4. To help students see the relevance of using visual characteristics to describe, pair students. Give each pair an object to describe and a *Visual Description* activity page. (Tell the pairs to keep their

objects a secret.) Have each pair use the *Creature Creator* poster to help them describe the size, shape, color, and distinctive feature of their object. Have each pair write their descriptions on the *Visual Description* activity page, then take turns reading their description for the rest of the class to guess what they are describing. Analyze communication breakdowns if they occur.

CLOSURE

Summarize the lesson, repeat its relevance to the students, and tie it to future learning. Have students think of when they might have to describe the characteristics of something (e.g., if you need something but do not know what it's called, describing its characteristics will help someone know what you want). Stress that communicating ideas clearly is a valuable lifelong tool. Tell students that in the next lesson they will use all five senses to describe different objects.

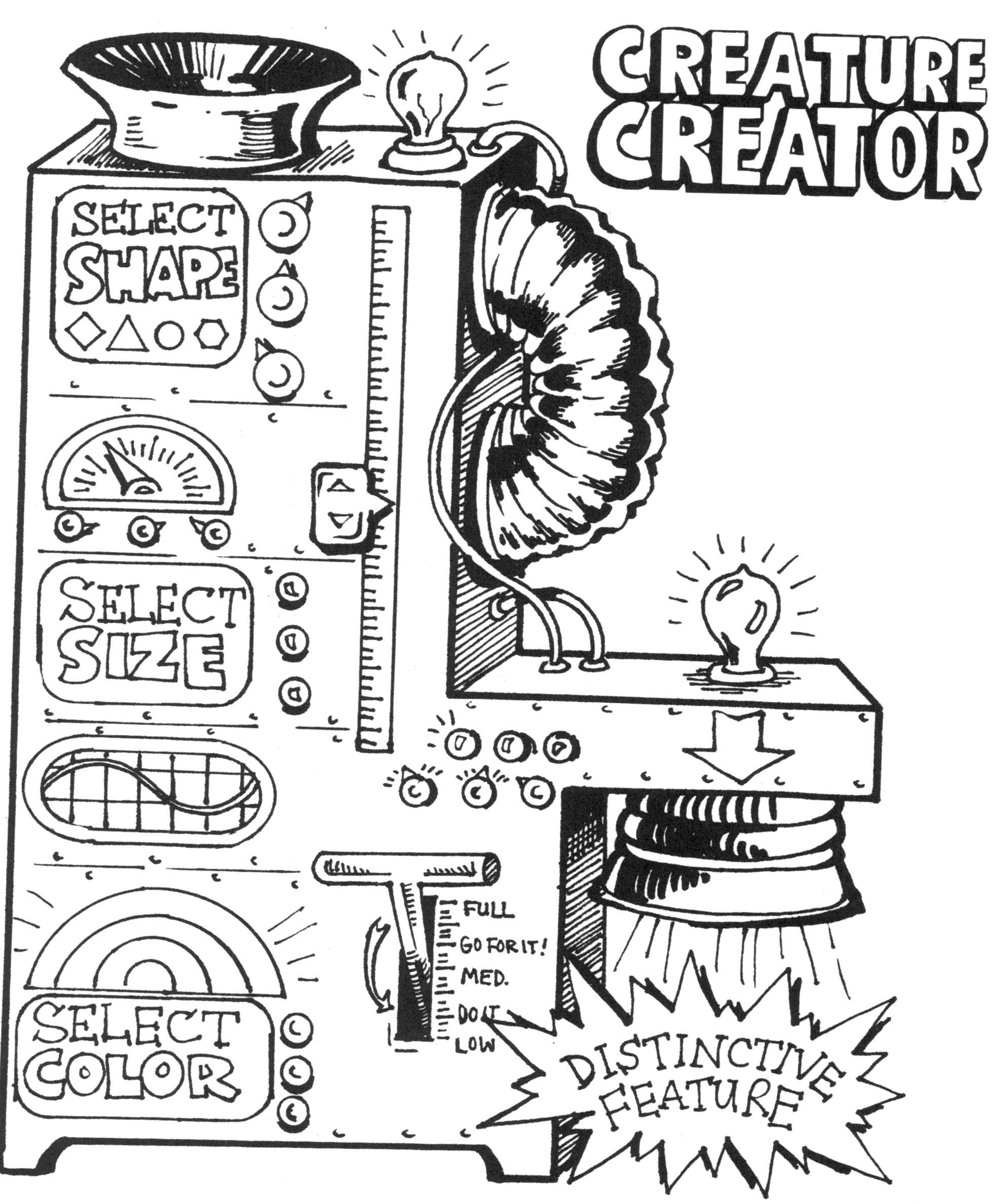
CREATURE CREATOR
SELECT SHAPE
SELECT SIZE
SELECT COLOR
FULL
GO FOR IT!
MED.
DO IT
LOW
DISTINCTIVE FEATURE

Weird Creature Parts

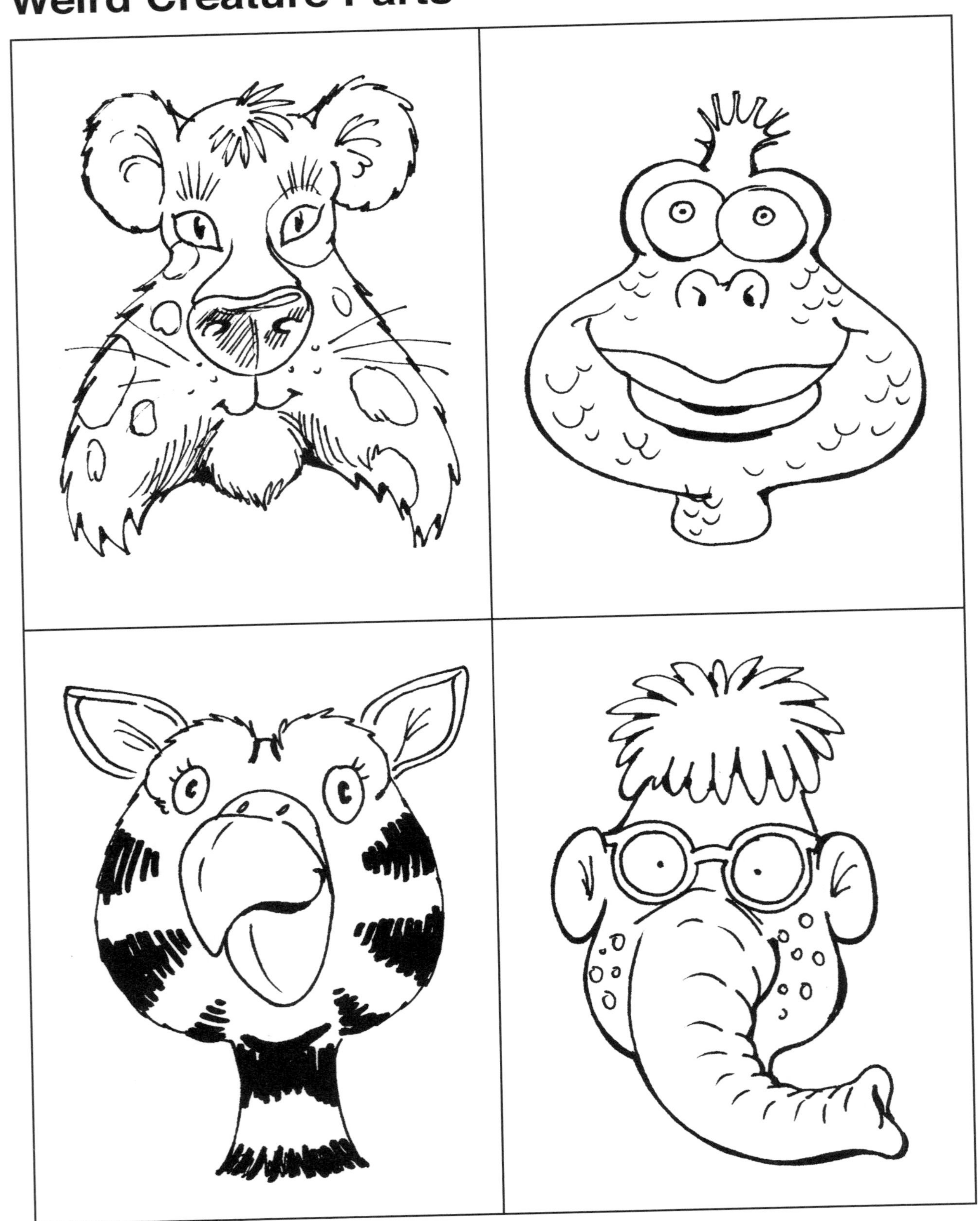

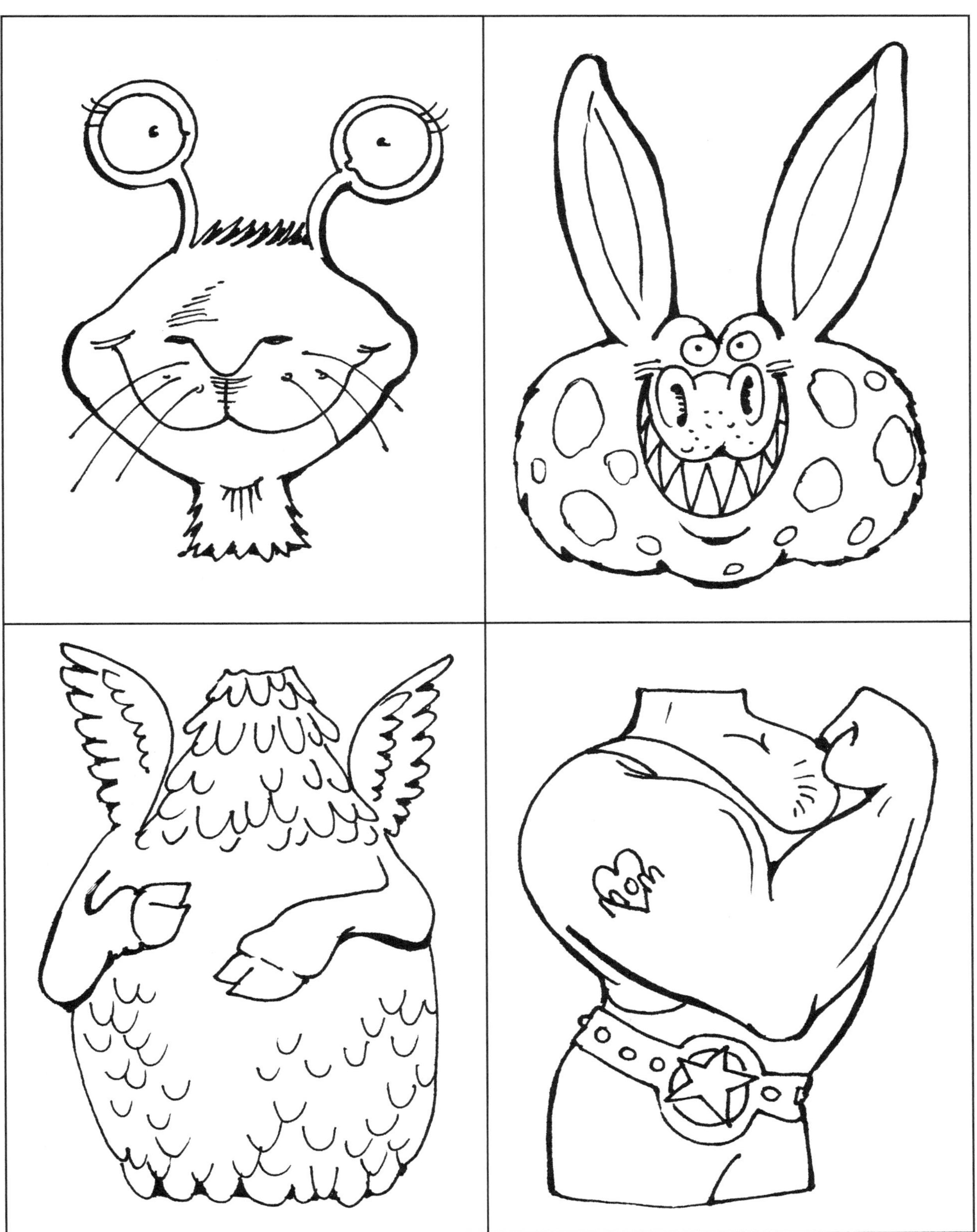
Mom

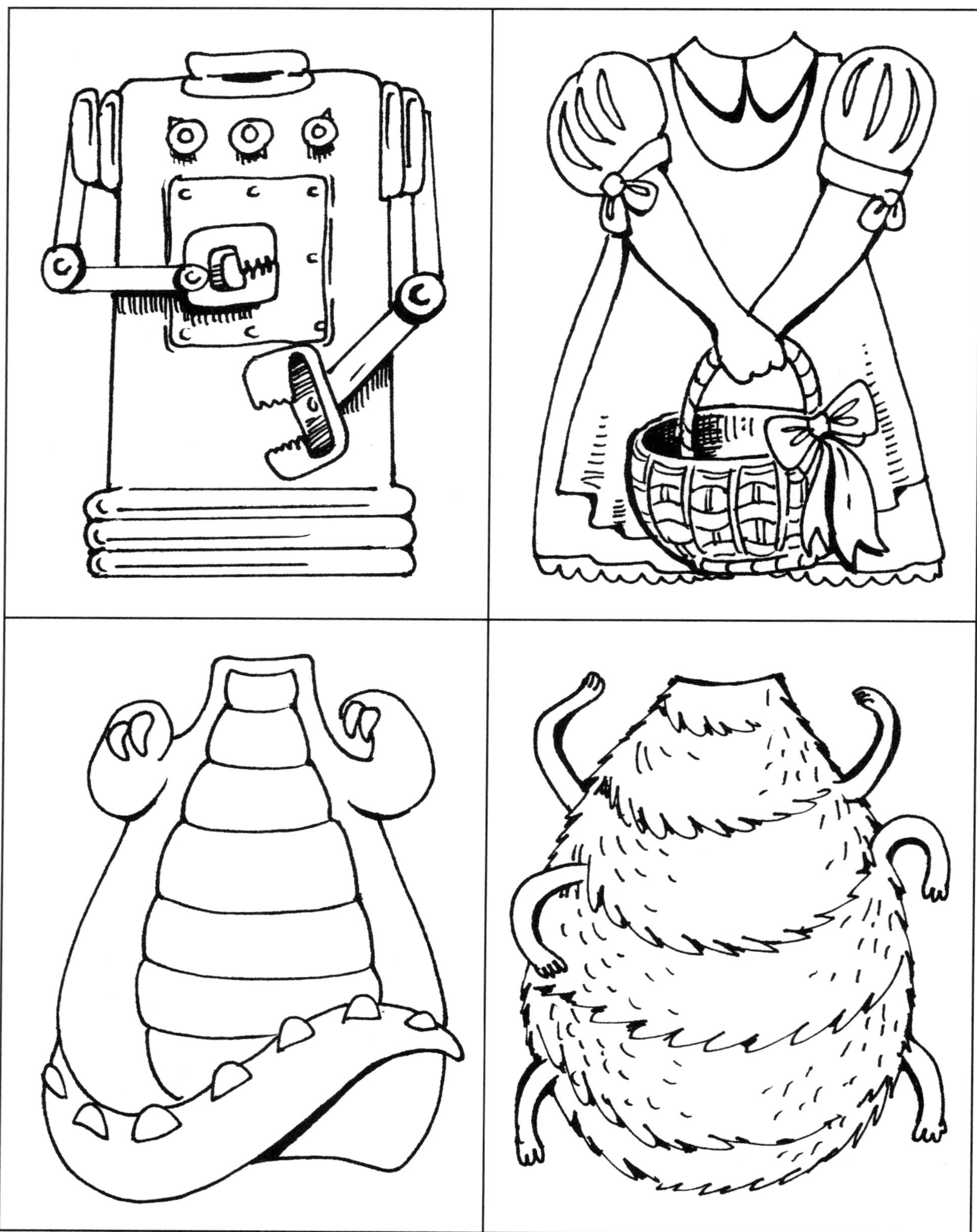

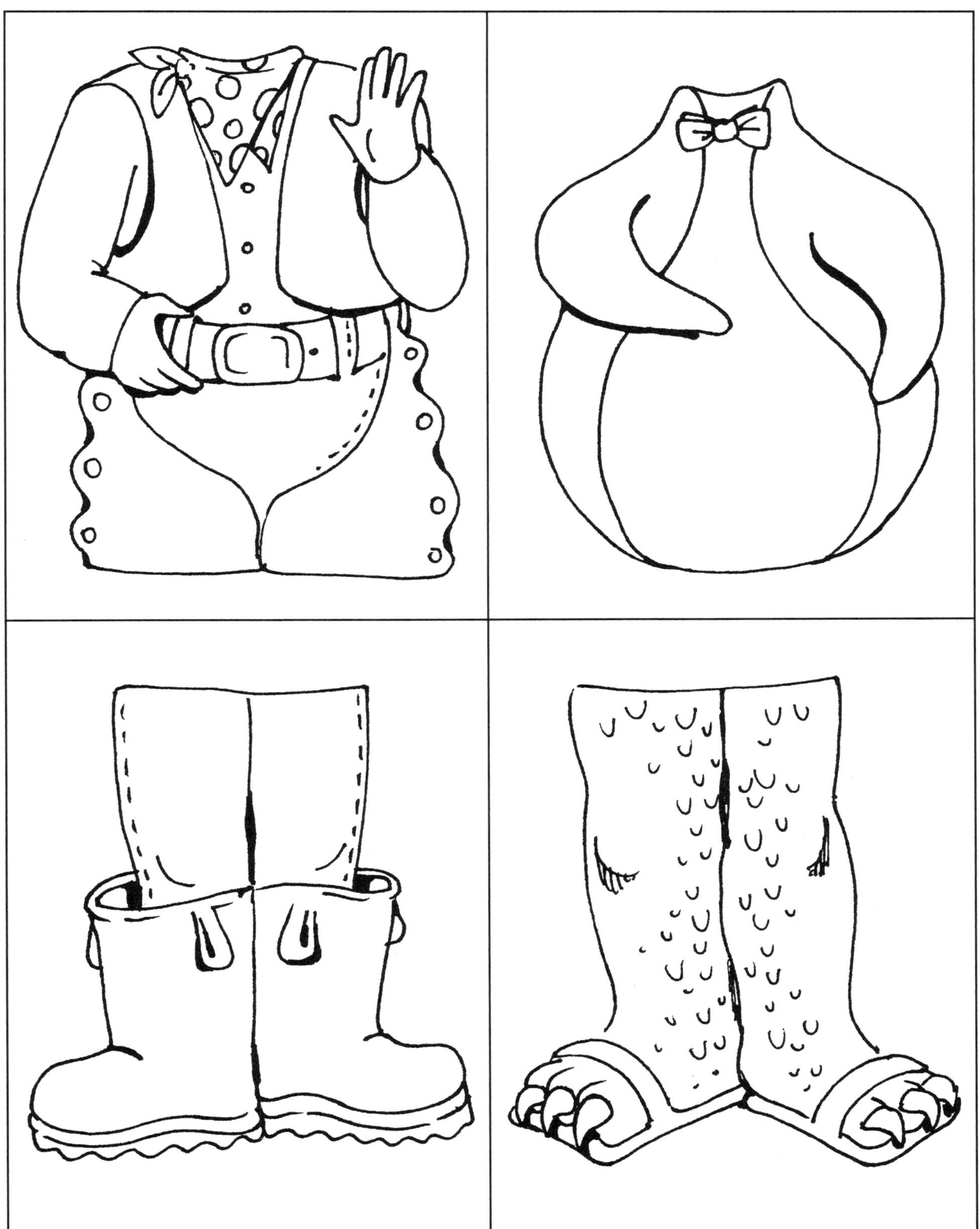

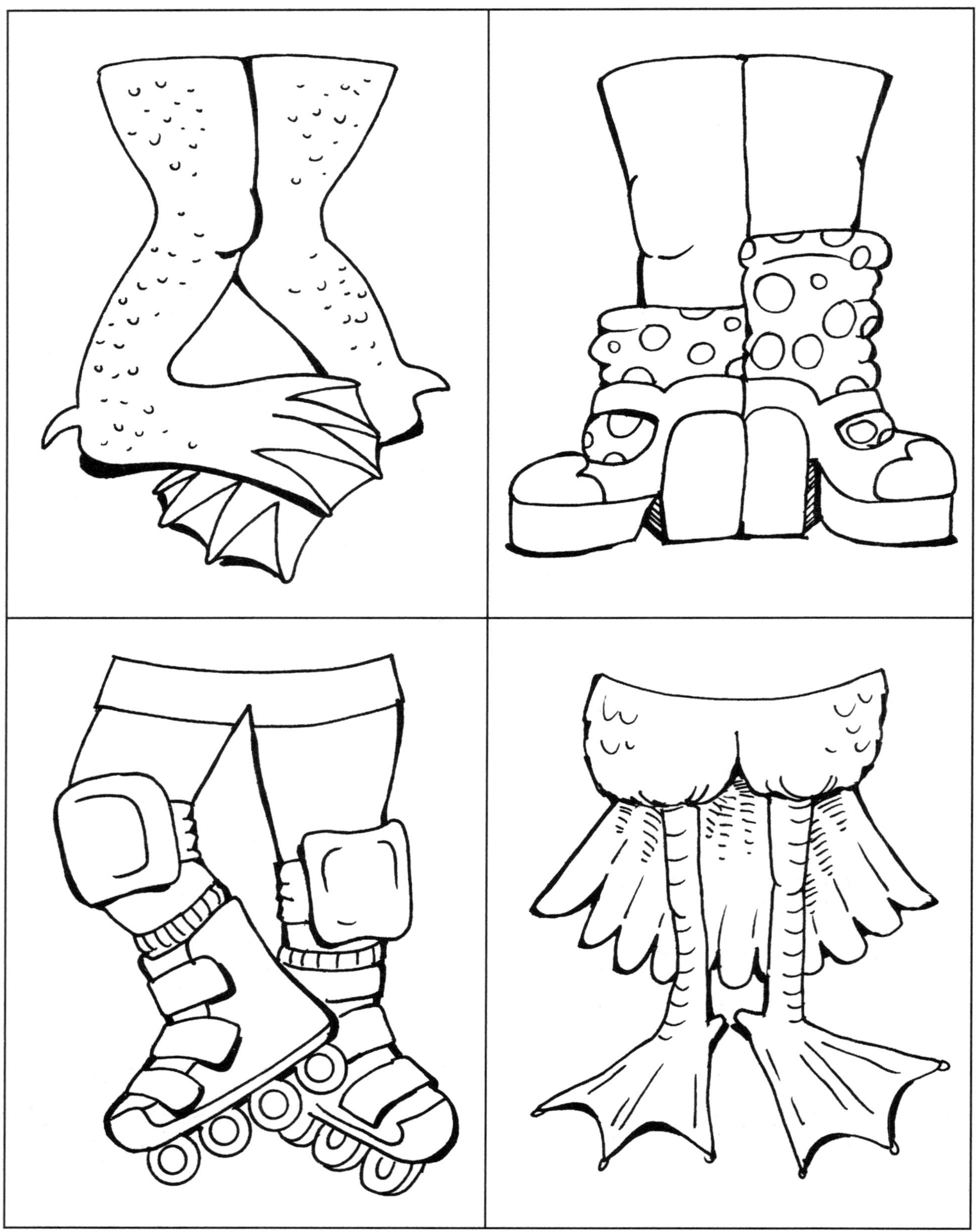

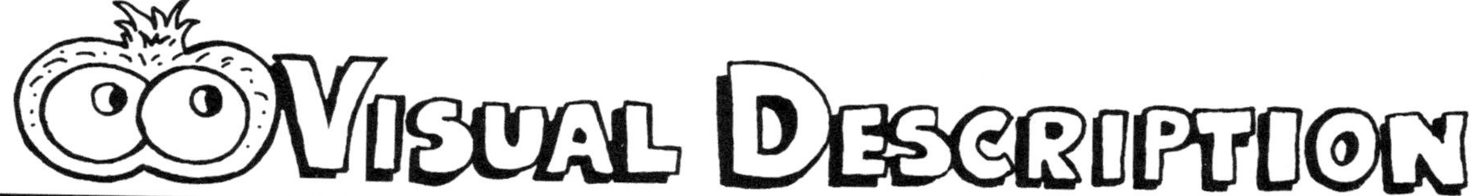

Name: ______________________________ Date: ______________

Directions: Describe the size, shape, color, and distinctive features of the item you are describing. Then write a one- or two-sentence description of it.

Size: ______________________________

____

Shape: ______________________________

____

Color: ______________________________

____

Distinctive Feature(s): ______________________________

____

____

____

Description: ______________________________

____

____

____

____

IT MAKES SENSE: DESCRIBING USING FIVE SENSES (PART I)

GOAL

To use precise descriptors in expressive language

BACKGROUND INFORMATION

The *It Makes Sense* strategy continues the work of building vocabulary knowledge and flexibility in word use started during the *Creature Creator* strategy. Students use size, shape, color, and distinctive feature characteristics to describe items. Information gathered using other senses is emphasized in this lesson and the next. Students still use attributes that are visually observable although the attribute might also fit another sense (e.g., a fuzzy attribute can be seen and felt).

OBJECTIVES

1. Name the five senses using the *It Makes Sense* strategy.
2. Use the five senses to describe objects.

MATERIALS

1. *It Makes Sense* graphic (See page 97; duplicate and enlarge the graphic, color it, mount it onto poster board, and laminate it for durability, if desired.)
2. Marshmallows (One per student)
3. Chalkboard and chalk
4. Other food items that can be contrasted with the marshmallows (e.g., pretzels, crackers)

INTRODUCTION

Tie-in to Prior Learning

Remind students that in the last lesson they learned how to describe items using visual attributes. Have students name the four characteristics that were used in previous descriptions (i.e., shape, size, color, and distinctive features). Review the meaning of *distinctive features*. Ask what would happen if you asked the student wearing tennis shoes to stand up. Ask, "Is this characteristic a distinctive feature in this classroom?"(Most likely this is not a distinctive feature because the majority of students might be wearing tennis shoes.) Then ask what would happen if you asked the student with (name a unique item worn by only one student in the class [e.g., the pink bow]) to stand. Remind students that a distinctive feature is a unique characteristic when compared to other members of the group. Have students give other examples of the unique features of objects or of students in the classroom.

Focus/Relevancy

Say to the students,

> *Today we're going to practice describing using all of our senses, not just our eyes. How could using all of your senses help you describe things more precisely?* (Write a simple sentence on the board [e.g., I ate an apple]. Read the sentence, act out a huge yawn.) *B-O-R-I-N-G! How can we make this sentence more descriptive?* (Students will find humor in this introduction and the point will be made. Take suggestions from the class for revising the sentence [e.g., "I ate the crisp, red apple"]). *After we practice describing using all of our senses, we can make this sentence even more interesting and descriptive. Describing something with precise words is a very important skill at school because use of descriptive words will help others know exactly what you mean and will help your speaking and writing be more interesting.*

LESSON ACTIVITIES

1. Put your hand on your face so that each finger touches a sense organ (i.e., your thumb on your ear, your index finger on your eye, your middle finger on your nose, your ring finger on your mouth, and your little finger on your chin to indicate touch). Ask students what this gesture might represent and encourage them to name the five senses (i.e., hearing, vision, smell, taste, and touch). Students may name the sense organs (e.g., eyes, ears, nose). Be sure to clarify the difference between the tools (i.e., the sense organs) for using our senses and the actual sense. The senses are what we do with our sense organs. Show the *It Makes Sense* poster. Explain that this strategy will aid the student in not only remembering the senses, but reminding them to use all their senses when describing. Model the use of sense words to describe a piece of chewing gum (e.g., "The pink chewing gum was sticky and sweet and popped when it formed a bubble").

2. Have the students pretend to be a group of scientists who have discovered the marshmallow. Although it has already been tested to determine that it is not poisonous, more observational detail is needed to really describe this "find." Discuss what the students need to know to describe this piece of "matter." Say,

   > *Let's see how many ideas we can think of that describe this strange substance. We will organize our ideas so that we can share them with scientists from around the world. What information should we share?*

3. Draw a chart on the board with a column for each of the five senses. Give the *It Makes Sense* signal and have the students name the five senses. Distribute one marshmallow to each student telling the class that they each have a sample of the "substance" to describe. Suggest students

begin with the sense of vision since it will provide a lot of information without damaging the sample. Ask the students what would happen to the scientist who begins with the sense of taste (e.g., he or she might have nothing left to observe).

4. Have the class brainstorm descriptions of the marshmallow considering the characteristics of size, shape, color, and distinctive feature while using only the sense of vision. Write responses on the chart. Summarize what has been discussed and ask if there are any other descriptions before moving on to each sense. There should be at least two descriptions for each sense.

   Vision—Use the *Creature Creator* poster as a reminder of visual characteristics to consider.

   Hearing—Objects by themselves may not make a noise; explain that the students may need to manipulate the marshmallow in some way (e.g., squish it or tap it) just as a scientist would experiment with the substance he or she has discovered.

   Touch—Remind students that the sense of touch is not just connected to the fingers (e.g., you can feel the wind on your face or the heat on your body when standing beside a hot stove).

   Taste and Smell—These senses are related. If an item smells sweet, it will most likely taste sweet. These senses could be combined on the chart.

5. The process can be repeated using a pretzel or some other contrasting food item. After brainstorming descriptive details, compare and contrast the two objects. For example, discuss the difference between salty and sweet. This can be a difficult concept for many students.

   HINT
   As an option, divide the group into two or more groups or teams of "scientists" to work independently. Relate this process to the way scientists search for new information and then share their findings. Have each group share their findings (i.e., their descriptions) with the group.

CLOSURE

Summarize the lesson, review its relevance to students, and tie it to future learning. Return to the original sentence (e.g., I ate an apple). Remind students that the lesson began with a very boring sentence that could be made interesting (spicy) by using senses. Use the chart described in step 3 to describe an apple. Elicit sense words from the chart to insert and revise the sentence. An example of a "spicy" sentence that may result as students now give descriptive words from all senses might be, "The shiny, smooth, red apple was sweet, juicy, and crunchy and had a little brown bruise on one side." Compare the new sentence to the original. Students are typically amazed at how dramatically they are able to revise the sentence.

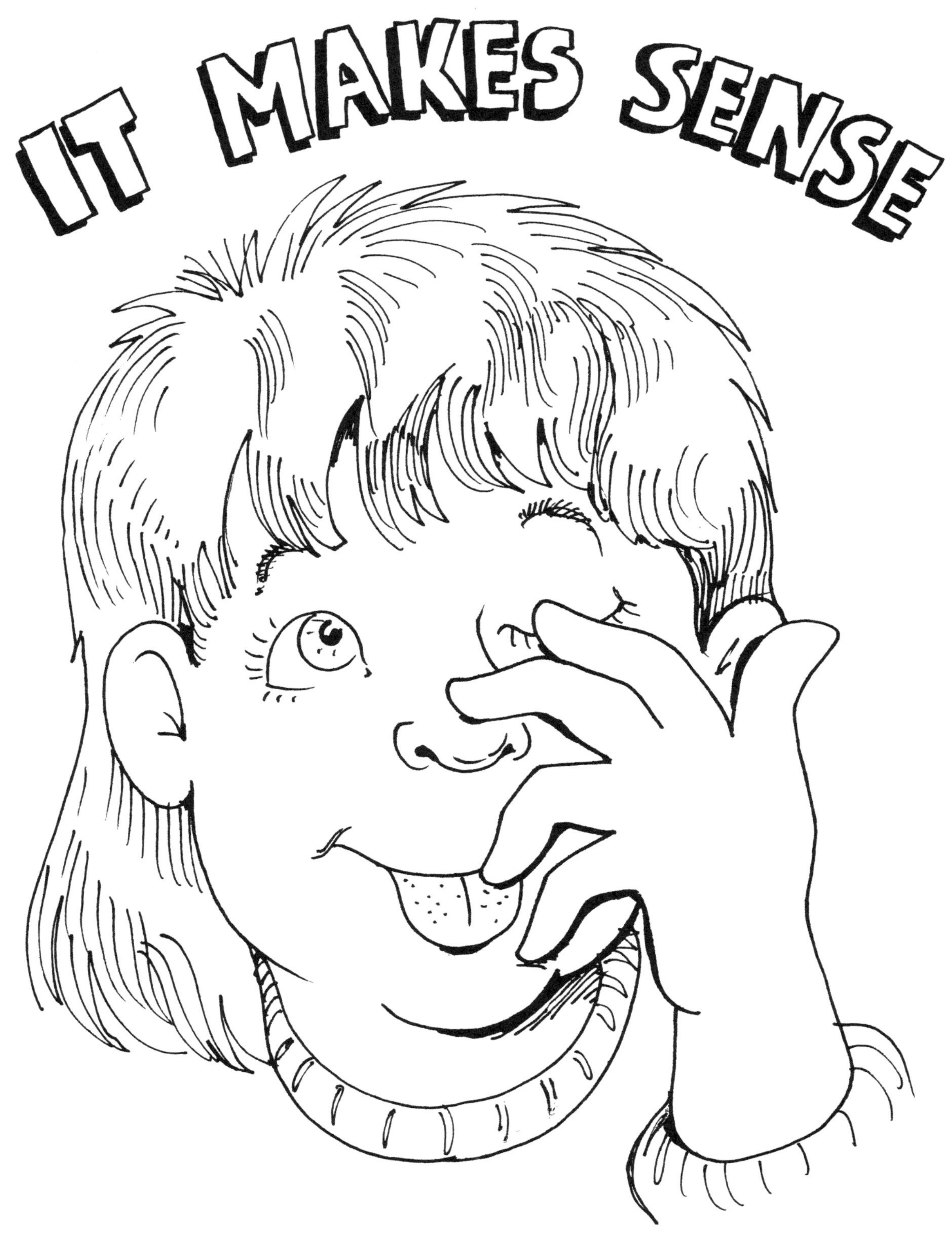
IT MAKES SENSE

IT MAKES SENSE: DESCRIBING USING FIVE SENSES (PART II)

GOAL

To use precise descriptors in expressive language

BACKGROUND INFORMATION

The *It Makes Sense* strategy continues the work of building vocabulary knowledge and flexibility in word use started during the *Creature Creator* strategy. Students use size, shape, color, and distinctive feature characteristics to describe items. Information gathered using other senses is emphasized in this lesson. Students still use attributes that are visually observable although the attribute might also fit another sense (e.g., a fuzzy attribute can be seen and felt).

OBJECTIVES

1. Name the five senses and use sensory words to describe objects.
2. Use descriptive words in sentences.
3. Learn the rules of sentence combining using *and.*

MATERIALS

1. *It Makes Sense* poster (Created earlier)
2. Assorted objects for describing (e.g., pine cones, seashells; one per group)
3. *Sense Chart* (See pages 101–102; duplicate one per group.)
4. *Five Senses Flip Book* (See pages 104–110; create one as an example following instructions on page 103; duplicate one set of pages per group.)

INTRODUCTION

Tie-in to Prior Learning

Remind students that in the last lesson they used more than just visual observations to describe objects. Ask a student to demonstrate the *It Makes Sense* strategy which reminds students to use five senses when describing. Refer to the *It Makes Sense* poster.

Focus/Relevancy

1. Introduce the lesson by saying to the students,

   We're going to continue sharpening our descriptive skills, but we want to make describing a little more challenging than in the last lesson. In addition to using interesting, descriptive sentences, we're also going to practice joining a number of details into one complete sentence.

2. Remind students that if they do not accurately describe what they want, they may not like what they get.

LESSON ACTIVITIES

1. Divide students into learning groups of three or four students each. Direct students to assign two roles within the group: a) a recorder to document the ideas (i.e., write them down); and b) a reporter to share the findings (i.e., the ideas) with the entire class at the end of the activity. All group participants are observers.

2. Distribute to each group a pine cone (or any object that might complement a curriculum concept) and a *Sense Chart.* Tell them that, as in the last lesson, they are again to pretend they are scientists who will be observing a substance. Direct the "scientists" in each group to study their object, observe the characteristics of the object using the five senses, and then document their findings on the *Sense Chart.* Tell students to write descriptive words and ideas for each sense on the chart. Encourage everyone in the group to contribute an idea. Explain that after brainstorming, they will decide on their most descriptive words to transfer to a flip book. Allow the students 5 to 10 minutes to complete the chart. Then have the reporter from each group share the group's findings.

   HINT
   Suggest that if the object cannot be tasted, students can predict what they think it might taste like. Remind students that taste and smell are related senses. What does it smell like to them? Do they think it might taste like it smells? For example, the pine cone might smell like a tree, so it might taste like wood. The students could base their predictions on prior experiences of knowing the taste of a popsicle stick.

3. Show the example of a completed *Five Senses Flip Book.* Explain that each group will be transferring their most descriptive ideas for each sense to a *Five Senses Flip Book.* On the last page is a pattern for combining ideas. Discuss the rules for using commas and conjunctions to combine ideas:

   a. When combining just two ideas, use the word *and.*

      Example: The pine cone is brown and bumpy.

   b. When listing more than two ideas, find the information that is redundant and draw lines through it. Rewrite the sentences into one shorter, more efficient sentence. Add commas to separate each ides and use *and* before the last idea.

Example: The pine cone is brown.
The pine cone is bumpy.
The pine cone has sharp points.

The pine cone is brown, bumpy, and has sharp points.

5. Discuss the reasons for combining several sentences into one sentence. Stress that students will not have to write as much if they combine ideas into one sentence. And the ideas will be more interesting to hear or read.

4. Distribute the flip book pages to each group and allow students time to complete them. Let each group share their flip books with the class. If desired, repeat this process with other objects related to a curriculum concept.

CLOSURE

Summarize the lesson, repeat its relevance to students, and tie it to future learning. Review rules for combining two or more ideas into a descriptive sentence. Start with a bland sentence and let the students suggest descriptive words to spice it up! Challenge the students to use their senses and observations when writing on their own. Have students think about other classes where being descriptive will help them be successful. Remind them to use the *It Makes Sense* strategy to help write an interesting description. Have students generate situations when they could apply the *It Makes Sense* strategy outside of school situations.

Names: ____________________

____

Sense Chart

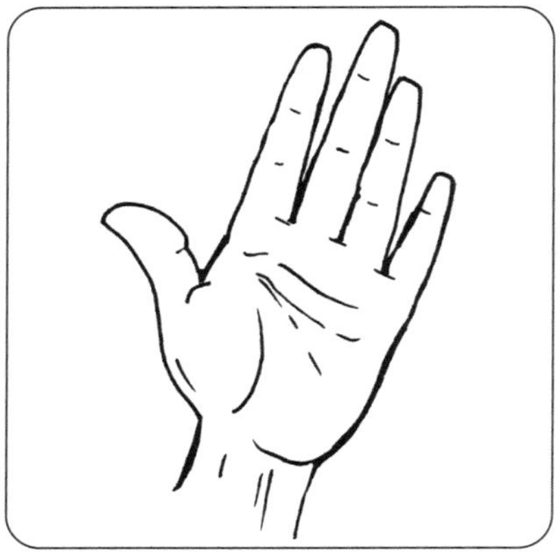

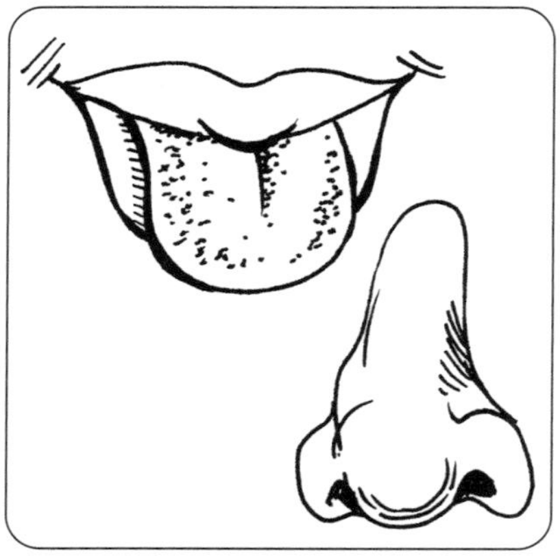

Directions for Creating Five Senses Flip Book

1. To create page A, use $8\frac{1}{2}$" x 14" paper to duplicate and enlarge (at 150%) pages A_1, A_2, and A_3. Run A_1 and A_2 back to back. Run A_3 at the bottom of A_1 as follows:

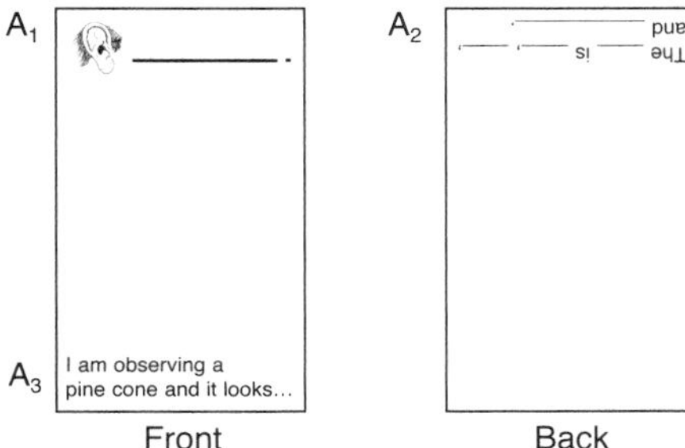

2. Duplicate and enlarge (at 118%) pages B front and back and C front and back on standard $8\frac{1}{2}$" x 11" paper.

3. Take one of each A, B, and C and arrange as follows:

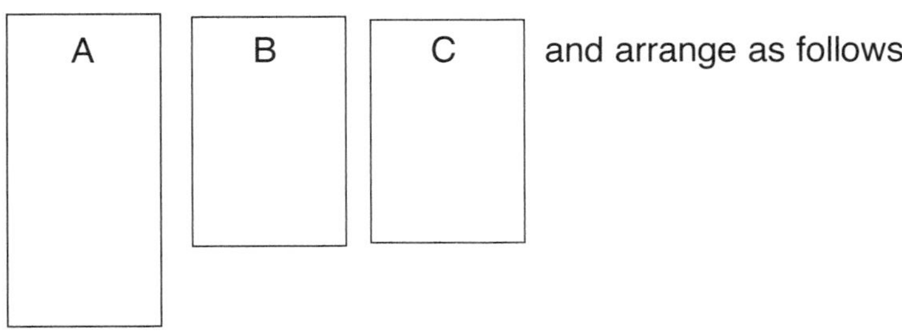

a. Stack A, B, and C.

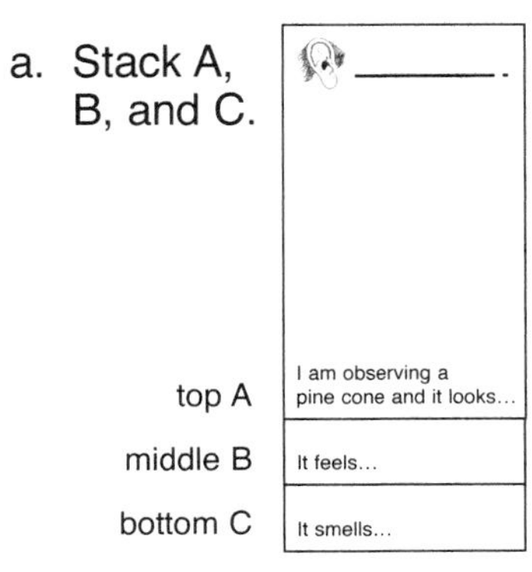

b. Pick up by the sides and fold as shown.

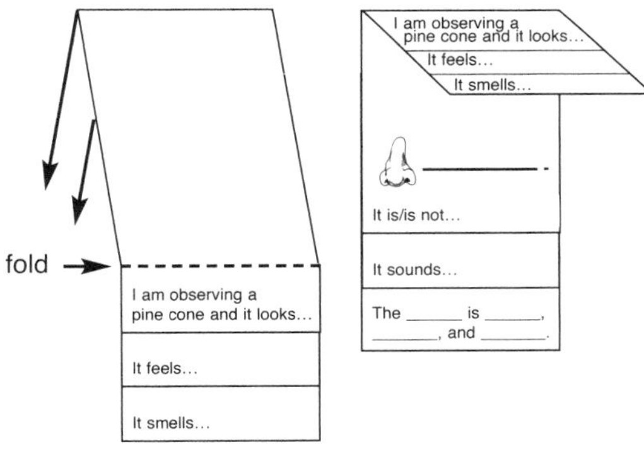

c. Staple.

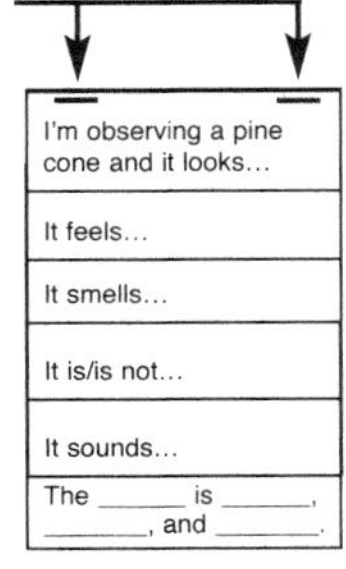

d. Fold bottom flap up and tuck under the "It sounds..." flap.

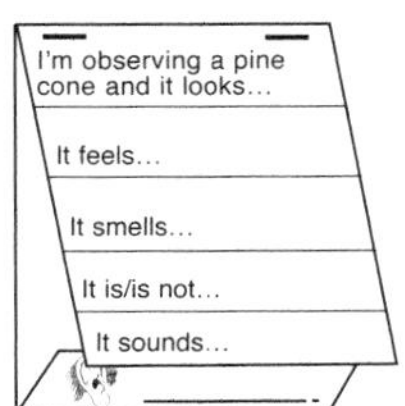

A_1 front

A_2
top back of A

The ______________ is ______________,
______________, and ______________.

A_3
bottom front of A

I am observing a pine cone and it looks...

B front

______________________________ .

It feels...

B back

Something I would taste. I predict it *might* taste like a ____.

It sounds…

C front

______________________________.

It smells...

C back

It is/ is not...

____.

CREATURE CREATOR and IT MAKES SENSE FOLLOW-UP ACTIVITIES

GOAL

To reinforce and review *Creature Creator* and *It Makes Sense* strategies

BACKGROUND INFORMATION

The main focus of this lesson is to review the previous two strategies. The strategy guide review pages will be compiled with other similar pages into a booklet. This booklet, along with a vacation calendar, provides a means of practicing with family members and reinforcing skills throughout a school break. Although some educators may choose to do the strategy guide pages and homework activities at the end of each lesson, others prefer delayed reinforcement to strengthen knowledge of strategies, concepts, and vocabulary covered within the lessons. Using a small representation of the strategy poster, the strategy guide pages include the specific vocabulary from the lessons. An application component is provided on the second pages of the strategy guides. Students may do reflective writing about how the strategy is or can be useful to them.

OBJECTIVES

1. Tell and write the major components of the *Creature Creator* and *It Makes Sense* strategies.
2. Reflect and write about how the strategies will help at home, at school, and in the community.
3. Share strategy information with family members and complete the application activities.

MATERIALS

1. *Creature Creator* poster (Created earlier)
2. *It Makes Sense* poster (Created earlier)
3. *Creature Creator Strategy Guide* (See pages 113–114; duplicate one per student.)
4. *It Makes Sense Strategy Guide* (See pages 115–116; duplicate one per student.)
5. *Creature Creator Homework Activity* (See page 117; duplicate one per student.)
6. *It Makes Sense Homework Activity* (See page 118; duplicate one per student.)

INTRODUCTION

Tie-in to Prior Learning

Remind students that they have now learned two more strategies that will help them move toward achieving their goals to improve describing skills. Display and review the posters and strategies for these lessons. Have students tell about each of the strategies in their own words.

Focus/Relevancy

Review the importance of the *Strategy Guide Booklet* which will be a collection of the student's strategy guide pages for each strategy learned. The booklet will help them become better communicators by helping them remember all the strategies they will be learning. Remind students that new pages are added as new strategies are learned. Say to them,

> *We're ready to add the next pages to our* Strategy Guide Booklet *to help remember the important strategies we've learned and how we might use the strategies every day.*

LESSON ACTIVITIES

1. Distribute the *Creature Creator Strategy Guide* pages and the *It Makes Sense Strategy Guide* pages and have students complete them. Students are to demonstrate they know the strategies by completing the blank lines.

2. On the second page of each strategy guide, have students write how each particular strategy has helped them or will help them at school, at home, or in the community. Brainstorm ideas (e.g., "I wanted to tell my Mom about a movie I saw. I thought about the *It Makes Sense* strategy and the strategy helped me to describe the movie better so she knew exactly what I saw," "In art class, we were supposed to draw a fun monster. The *Creature Creator* strategy helped me plan what I would draw"). Have students brainstorm other ways they might apply the strategy and then write how they will apply the strategy on their strategy guide pages.

3. Hand out the *Creature Creator* and the *It Makes Sense Homework Activity* pages and discuss them. Reinforce the importance of sharing this information with family members, and the ease and fun of doing these assignments. They will only take a few minutes to complete, but students can impress their family with what they have learned! Have a reward system established to encourage students to bring their homework activity pages back to school signed by a family member.

CLOSURE

Summarize the lesson, review its relevance to students, and tie it to future learning. Discuss the objectives that were completed in this review (i.e., the students can tell and write the *Creature Creator* and *It Makes Sense* strategies; they can tell how they will use the strategies; they know the strategies well enough to share them with their family members).

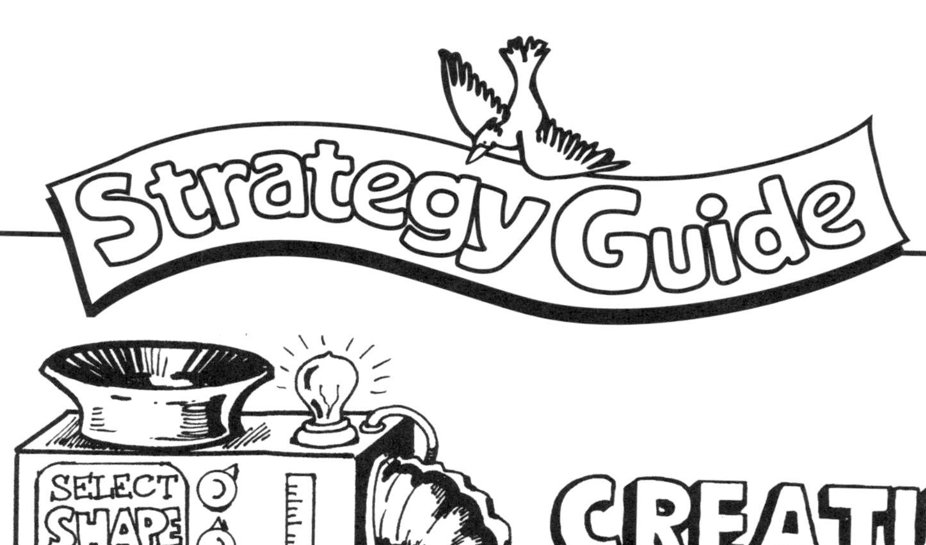

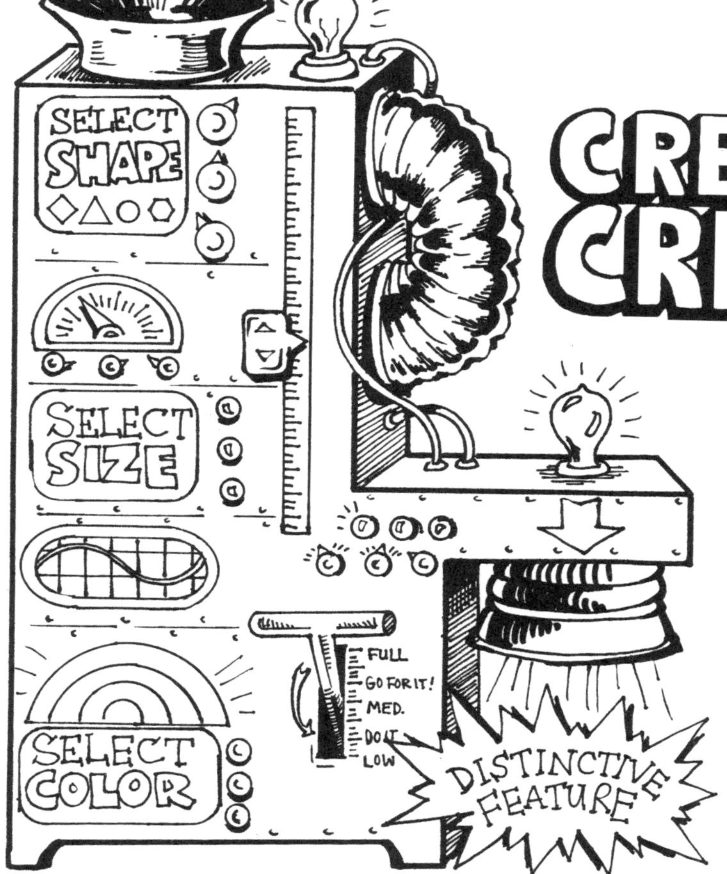

Describe an egg:

1. ______________________________

2. ______________________________

3. ______________________________

4. ______________________________

Creature Creator: Describing Using Vision

Name: ______________________ Date: ____________

Directions: Write a sentence about how you have used or will use the strategy in each place.

At home, I ______________________

____

____

____

____

____

At school, I ______________________

____

____

____

____

____

In my community, I ______________________

____

____

____

____

____

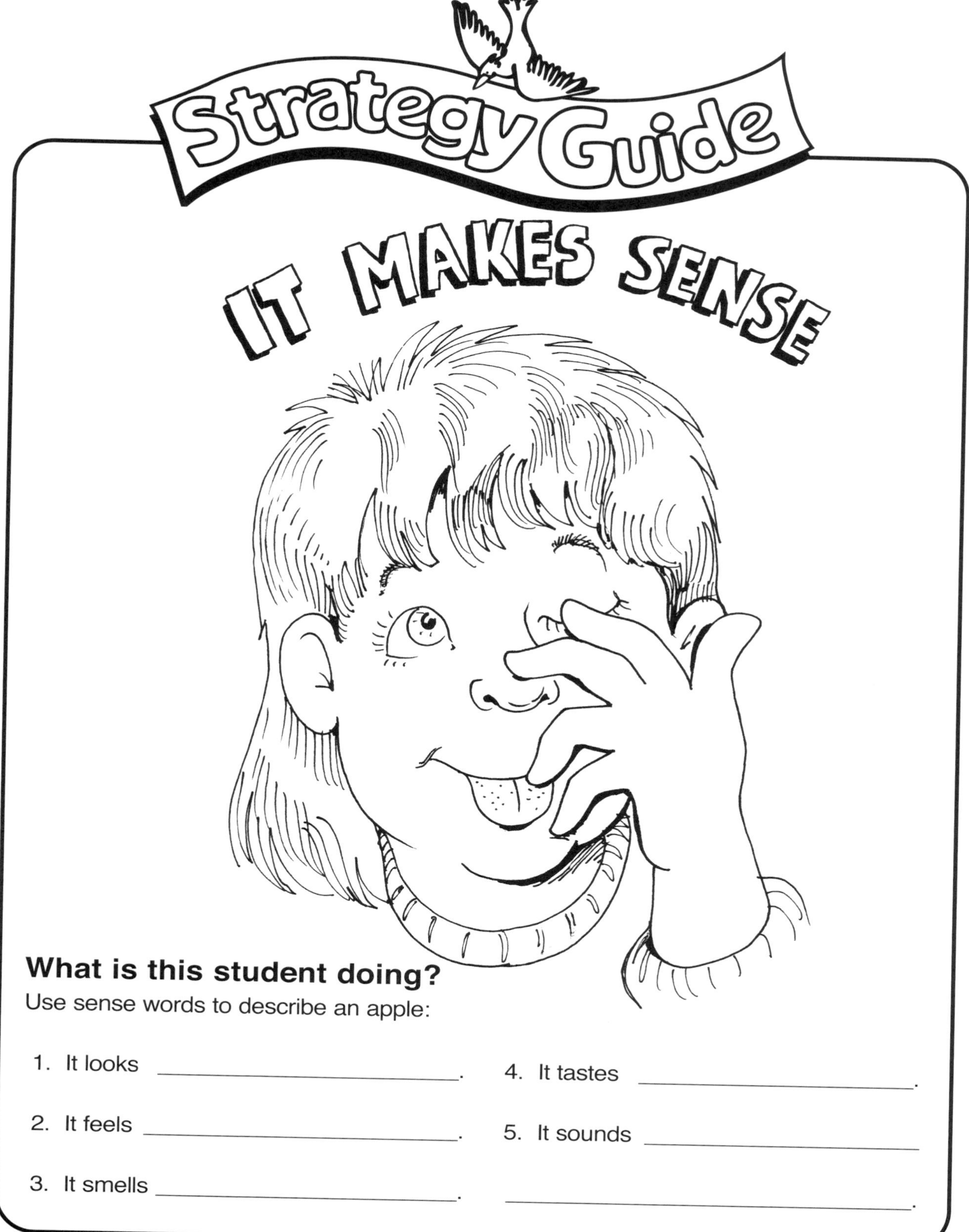

What is this student doing?

Use sense words to describe an apple:

1. It looks ______________________.
2. It feels ______________________.
3. It smells ______________________.
4. It tastes ______________________.
5. It sounds ______________________
______________________.

It Makes Sense: Describing Using Five Senses

Name: ______________________ Date: ____________

Directions: Write a sentence about how you have used or will use the strategy in each place.

At home, I ______________________________

____

____

____

____

____

At school, I ______________________________

____

____

____

____

____

In my community, I ______________________________

____

____

____

____

____

Homework Activity

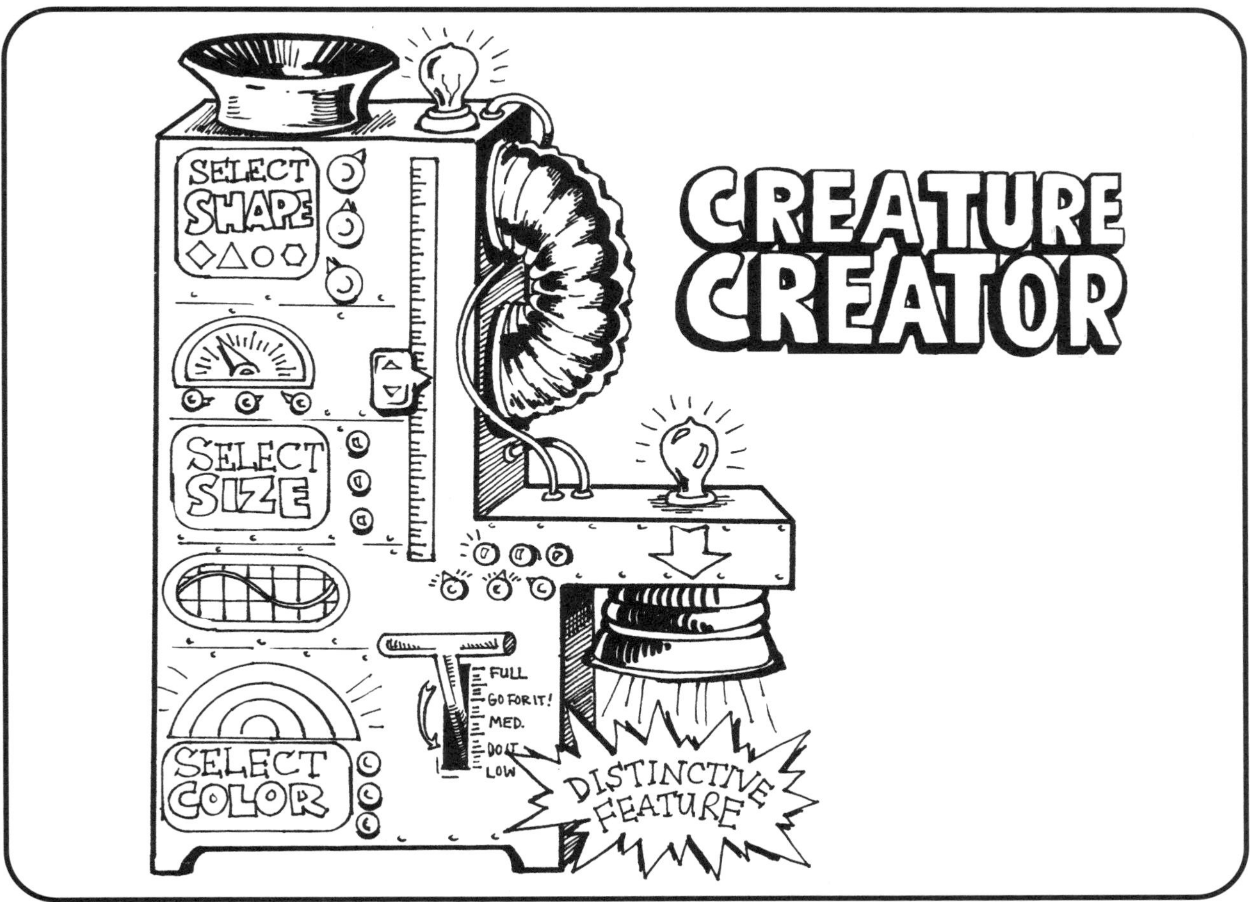

Dear Family,

1. Have your child explain the *Creature Creator* strategy and tell how it can help them be more descriptive.
2. Ask your child to tell a distinctive feature—something special or unique that sets him or her apart—about each member of your family.
3. Pick any object in your home and help your child use the *Creature Creator* strategy to describe it. The description should include shape, size, color, and distinctive features.
4. If your child completes these activities, please sign below and return this form to school.

Family Member: ______________________________________ Date: ______________

Homework Activity

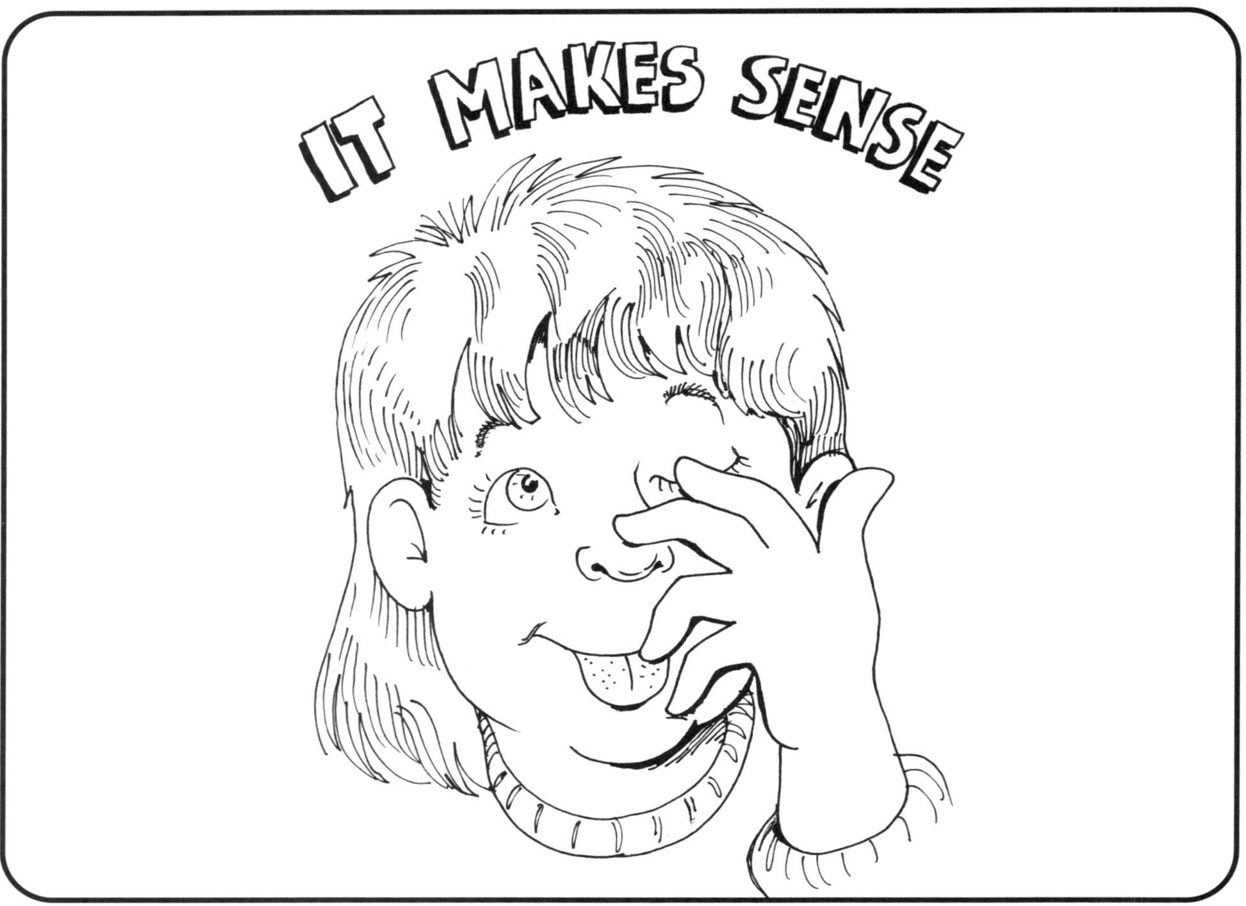

Dear Family,

1. Have your child explain the *It Makes Sense* strategy and tell how he or she can use the senses to be more descriptive.
2. Ask your child to use his or her senses to describe an ice cream cone that's being eaten by someone who is standing on a beach on a hot, sunny day.
3. Help your child describe a new bike he or she would like. Help him or her use all of the senses in the description.
4. If your child completes these activities, please sign below and return this form to school.

Family Member: ______________________________ Date: ____________

LASSO THE WORD HERD: CATEGORIZATION (PART I)

GOAL

To improve categorization skills

BACKGROUND INFORMATION

The *Lasso the Word Herd* strategy is part of a series of strategies that help students develop higher level thinking skills. The students will learn about describing attributes visually as well as with all five senses, categorizing, comparing and contrasting, and naming antonyms and synonyms. These lessons work to build vocabulary and flexibility in word knowledge and use.

Most of the world around us is organized into various categories. Grocery stores, department stores, parking lots, libraries, and cities are all organized by various types of attributes. If students understand the organizational systems (i.e., the systems for categorizing) used, they can be more efficient in understanding and later using a concept, system, or object. The foundation of categorization is recognizing similarities and differences. These next two lessons provide opportunities for grouping items, first by discussing similarities and then by discussing similarities and differences.

OBJECTIVE

1. Categorize by telling how members of a group are alike.

MATERIAL

1. *Roxaboxen* (1991) by Alice McLerran; Barbara Cooney, illustrator (If desired, substitute another book. *Roxaboxen* was chosen because it lends itself to discussions about organization within a community. The story is about a group of children growing up in the Arizona desert in the 1930s or 1940s. The children create a fantasy community out of old wooden boxes, rocks, and desert glass they find on a deserted hillside.)

INTRODUCTION

Tie-in to Prior Learning

Remind students that in the last lesson they learned to use all of their senses to generate descriptive words. Descriptive words help to make speaking and writing more interesting. Students can also use all of their senses in this lesson to help them discuss similarities and differences.

Focus/Relevancy

1. Before reading the story, *Roxaboxen,* highlight the literary components (see page 12). Discuss the author and illustrator. In addition, discuss the following:

- Cover—Tell students that this story probably takes place in the 1940s, and have them figure out mathematically how many years ago that would be.

- Rural versus urban—Ask students what games they think kids might have played at that time if they lived in a rural area. Discuss the difference between rural and urban areas and list the characteristics of each area. Relate the lists to the idea of organizing or categorizing groups that are alike in some way. For example, show the first illustration in the book which depicts a desert scene at sunset. Have the students list things that might be found in a desert (e.g., cactus, sand, snakes). Tell the students that they have now identified members of the category called "things found in a desert." Prepare the students for listening to the story by telling them that it will provide many ideas for categorizing. Say to the students,

  We created a category when we listed things found in a desert. Many school activities require us to group ideas or words together and to be able to justify or defend why we grouped them in a certain way. There is probably not a day that goes by that we do not have to categorize something.

2. Ask the students to think of activities during their day, whether at school, at home, or in the community that require categorizing or organizing (e.g., math involves grouping numbers by ones and tens; science involves grouping families of animals, or minerals; cleaning their rooms requires putting items in a particular place [games on shelves, toys in boxes, clothes in drawers]). Have students think of things that are not organized in some way. They should discover it is virtually impossible to do so.

LESSON ACTIVITIES

1. Read the story *Roxaboxen.* While reading the story, point out the following literary highlights:

   - Vocabulary—Define the words *pottery, general, mayor, scout, bandits, amber, amethyst, parlor,* and *bridle.*

   - Organization of a community—Discuss community concepts as they occur in the story. *Roxaboxen* contains the following categories that could be highlighted: buildings in a neighborhood, currency, goods and services, occupations, transportation, city government, rules and laws.

   - Multiple meaning words—Discuss how the words *ford, plain,* and *rock* are used in the story.

   - Real versus fiction—Before reading the one-page epilogue at the end of the story, ask how many students think that *Roxaboxen* is a true story. Why or why not? Then read the epilogue which explains how the story was based on old journals and stories passed on by the author's aunt. *Roxaboxen's* exact location in Yuma, Arizona is given.

2. After reading the story, point out the following literary highlights:
   - Epilogue—Talk about the importance of keeping a journal for future generations to know about our lifetime.

CLOSURE

Summarize the lesson, repeat its relevance to students, and tie it to future learning. Have the students list the kinds of community categories mentioned in the story and compare to how their own community is organized. Ask students to think of their classroom as their community. What categories do they observe in their classroom? Tell students that in the next lesson, they will play a game that will help strengthen their skills in categorizing.

LASSO THE WORD HERD: CATEGORIZATION (PART II)

GOAL

To improve categorization skills

BACKGROUND INFORMATION

The *Lasso the Word Herd* strategy is part of a series of strategies that help students develop higher level thinking skills. The students will learn about describing attributes visually as well as with all five senses, categorizing, comparing and contrasting, and naming antonyms and synonyms. These lessons work to build vocabulary and flexibility in word knowledge and use.

Most of the world around us is organized into various categories. Grocery stores, department stores, parking lots, libraries, and cities are all organized by various types of attributes. If students understand the organizational systems (i.e., the systems for categorizing) used, they can be more efficient in understanding and later using a concept, system, or object. The foundation of categorization is recognizing similarities and differences. This lesson provides opportunities for grouping items, first by discussing similarities and then by discussing similarities and differences.

OBJECTIVES

1. Categorize by telling how members of a group are alike.
2. Build flexibility in grouping words that fit into more than one category.

MATERIALS

1. *Lasso the Word Herd* graphic (See page 125; duplicate and enlarge the graphic, color it, mount it onto post board, and laminate it for durability, if desired.)
2. *Lasso the Word Herd* graphic (See page 125; create one overhead transparency.)
3. Overhead projector
4. Water soluble marker

INTRODUCTION

Tie-in to Prior Learning

Remind students about the special community in the story *Roxaboxen* that was read during the last lesson. Ask students to describe the community. Was it an urban or rural area? Have students defend their answers with facts from the story.

Focus/Relevancy

Show the *Lasso the Word Herd* poster and discuss how the lasso forms a circle for grouping words that are alike. Relate the strategy to a herd of cattle that are alike because they belong to the same farmer. Say to the students,

> *We produced a category when we listed parts of a desert. Many school activities require us to group ideas or words together and to be able to justify or defend why we grouped them in a certain way. Remember, there is probably not a day that goes by that we do not have to categorize something.* (Refer to *focus/relevancy* in Part I.)

LESSON ACTIVITIES

1. Display the *Lasso the Word Herd* transparency. Tell students they will be playing the game "In Crowd—Out Crowd." Explain the rules by saying,

> *One person will be the writer. The writer will think of a category but does not tell the group what it is. The writer will write one or two words from this category within the lasso on the transparency using the water color marker. These words will be part of the "in crowd," because they fit in the category. The rest of the group will try to guess words that they think are part of the "in crowd" without telling the actual category name. As each word is given, the writer will decide if the word is part of the "in crowd" or part of the "out crowd." If the word is part of the "in crowd," it will be written in the lasso circle. If the word is part of the "out crowd," it will be written outside of the lasso circle. For example, a player might see the words* apple, cherry, strawberry *inside the lasso and then guess the word* pear. *If the writer's category is red things, he or she will put the word* pear *outside of the circle. As more words are added either inside or outside of the circle, more of you will figure out the secret category. You will demonstrate this by giving additional words that fit within the category. Remember that the category name is a secret. You can show you know the answer by giving other words that fit the category. We will continue playing the game until no one is giving words that are part of the "out crowd" group or until we run out of room. Then the writer will share the secret category with the group.*

HINT

If the writer chooses a difficult category and the group has a difficult time discerning it, stop and summarize the information listed inside as well as outside of the lasso circle (e.g., "We know that *strawberries, apples,* and *cherries* are in the word herd, but that *pear* and *lettuce* are out of the word herd." Point to the items inside the lasso. "How are these items alike? Show me that you know the answer by telling another word that fits the category"). Or if students do not seem to know the category, the writer may need to add more examples within the lasso to help guide the players. Try to keep playing until everyone has figured it out. Have a player tell how the words inside the lasso are alike. Encourage them to use the wording such as, "They are alike because they are all _____."

2. Play the "In Crowd—Out Crowd" game using community-related categories (i.e., occupations, transportation, urban or rural) or any category ideas that support classroom curriculum concepts.

CLOSURE

Summarize the lesson, review its relevance to students, and tie it to future learning. Remind students that they have been practicing categorizing or grouping words together by playing the "In Crowd—Out Crowd" game and brainstorming members of a category. For these activities, they had to *compare* how words and ideas were alike or different. Have students think about how categorizing and organizing can help them be better students. In the next lesson, the students will learn another way to organize ideas when comparing and contrasting.

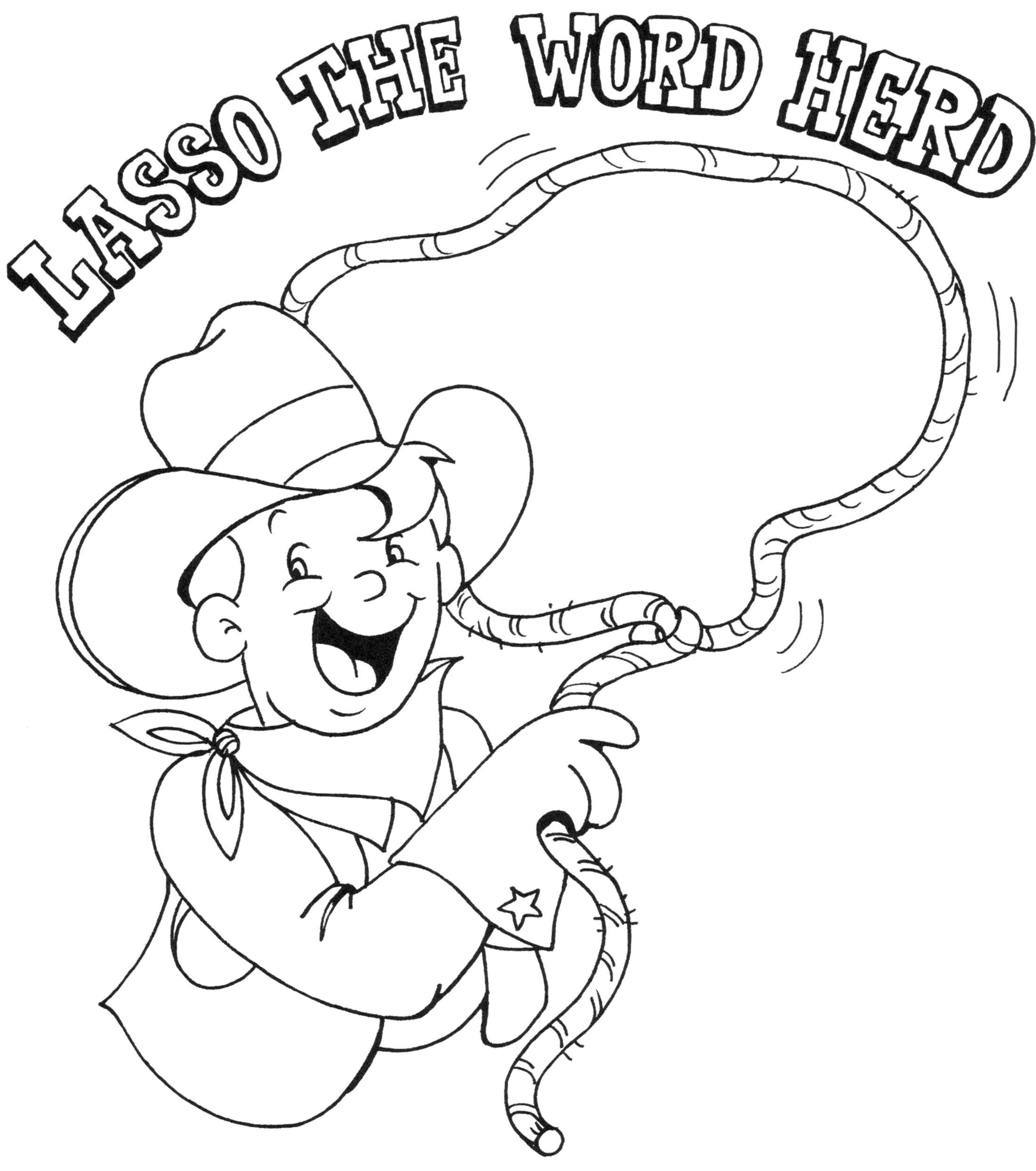
LASSO THE WORD HERD

COMPARE CONTRASTADON: COMPARING AND CONTRASTING

GOAL

To compare and contrast information

BACKGROUND INFORMATION

The *Compare Contrastadon* strategy is part of a series of strategies that help students develop higher level thinking skills necessary for solving analogies which includes: describing attributes visually as well as with all five senses, categorizing, comparing and contrasting, and naming antonyms and synonyms. These lessons work to build vocabulary and flexibility in word knowledge and use.

This lesson requires students to compare and contrast countries. This is an abstract activity that may be challenging for younger students. The activity can be simplified by using locations that are familiar to students such as one local town contrasted with another local town.

An optional curriculum tie-in would be to use a map of the United States (or Canada) to show the following sequence: country, state (or province), county (or other equivalent term, such as *parish*), city, town, neighborhood. Students may be chosen to stand with a card labeling each of the above. They could then rearrange themselves to be in ascending or descending order. Compare this to the use of a Venn diagram and encourage the use of a graphic organizer as a quick prewriting or thought-organizing strategy.

OBJECTIVES

1. Understand and use the terms *compare* and *contrast.*
2. Compare and contrast words, ideas, places, or events.

MATERIALS

1. *This Is My House* (1992) by Arthur Dorros (If desired, substitute another book. *This Is My House* was chosen because it describes homes or shelters in various parts of the world. The book also includes the phrase *This is my house* in each country's language with the pronunciation under it. It lends itself to comparing and contrasting geographic regions, natural resources, and sounds and symbols of different languages in a simple picture book format.)
2. *Compare Contrastadon* graphic (See page 130; duplicate and enlarge the graphic, color it, mount it onto poster board, and laminate it for durability, if desired.)
3. *Compare Contrastadon* graphic (See page 130; create one overhead transparency.)
4. Overhead projector
5. Water soluble marker

6. Small slips of paper with the names of countries (or locations) written on them and then folded (See step 5.)

INTRODUCTION

Tie-in to Prior Learning

Remind students that they have become expert thinkers and evaluators by practicing categorizing. Remind them that in the last lesson they played the category game "In Crowd—Out Crowd" and thought about how the words in the "word herd" were alike. Tell students that in this lesson, categorizing will be a little more challenging using the *Compare Contrastadon* strategy.

Focus/Relevancy

1. Introduce the *Compare Contrastadon* strategy by saying,

   You've heard of Tyrannosaurus rex and the pterodactyl dinosaurs but how many of you have heard of a compare contrastadon? What do you think it could be?

2. Display the *Compare Contrastadon* poster. Point out how the compare contrastadon has two heads and each is different. And the compare contrastadon's heads have one body in common. The body can be used to write how two things are alike and the heads (especially the neck portion) can be used to write the differences between two things or ideas.

3. Using the overhead transparency (or the poster, if laminated) and the water soluble marker, demonstrate a compare/contrast activity using simple concepts such as pizza and spaghetti, apples and oranges, or boots and tennis shoes. Write the concepts being compared to the right and left of the compare contrastadon's necks.

4. Have students brainstorm how the concepts are different and write the ideas on the corresponding necks. Tell students that when you contrast two things you are telling how they are different.

5. Then have students brainstorm how the concepts are similar and write the ideas on the compare contrastadon's body. Explain to students that when they are asked to compare, they are telling how words or ideas are alike.

LESSON ACTIVITIES

1. Before reading the story *This Is My House,* highlight the literary components (see page 12). Discuss the author and illustrator. In addition, discuss the following:

- Transportation—Discuss modes of transportation needed to travel to a location from one's home.

2. Read the story. (The entire book does not need to be read; specific locations may be selected for the purpose of this lesson.) While reading the story, point out the following literary highlights:

    - Geography—Identify each location on the map or globe as you read about it.

    - Vocabulary—Define the words *resources, shelter, desert, stilts, thatch, nomad, adobe, climate, pueblo, skyscraper, scaffolding, urban,* and *rural.*

3. After reading the story, point out the following literary highlights:

    - Shelter—Discuss vocabulary terms related to a community and varying resources available in the different locations. Why did the people in the location choose their particular type of shelter?

    - Vocabulary—Discuss map and globe terms or discuss environmental and weather-related terms (e.g., *climate, elevation).*

4. Have students compare their home town and state (or province) with a location in the book using the *Compare Contrastado*n transparency. Choose a location and write it on one side of the graphic and write the students' home town on the other side. Brainstorm with students ways that the two locations are different and record the differences on the appropriate neck of the compare contrastadon. Again brainstorm with students the ways the two locations are similar and write their responses on the compare contrastadon's body.

5. Repeat this exercise with other countries mentioned in *This Is My House.* Have two students each pick a slip of paper with the names of the countries (or other locations) mentioned in the book. With the book as a reference source, help students compare and contrast the two countries using the transparency. Encourage students to list several differences and several similarities. As they write each similarity or difference, encourage students to use a complete sentence to describe the relationship (e.g., "They are alike because they are both _______. They are different because one has__________ and the other…").

6. Demonstrate a more practical use for the *Compare Contrastadon* strategy by showing students how useful listing pros and cons can be for making decisions (e.g., deciding whether to buy a new baseball cap with your allowance money or to go to a movie with your friend). Discuss how comparing and contrasting is the basis for all decisions we make. Have students brainstorm other examples.

CLOSURE

Summarize the lesson, review its relevance to students, and tie it to future learning. Remind students that by using some type of strategy like *Compare Contrastadon*, they will be able to organize their ideas before making decisions, or before speaking or writing. It will also help them remember information in an organized way. Have students brainstorm situations in school where they are asked to compare and contrast ideas or concepts. Challenge them to give an example from every subject area (e.g., in science, when learning about different animals; in social studies, when learning about different time periods; in reading, when talking about different books and their characters).

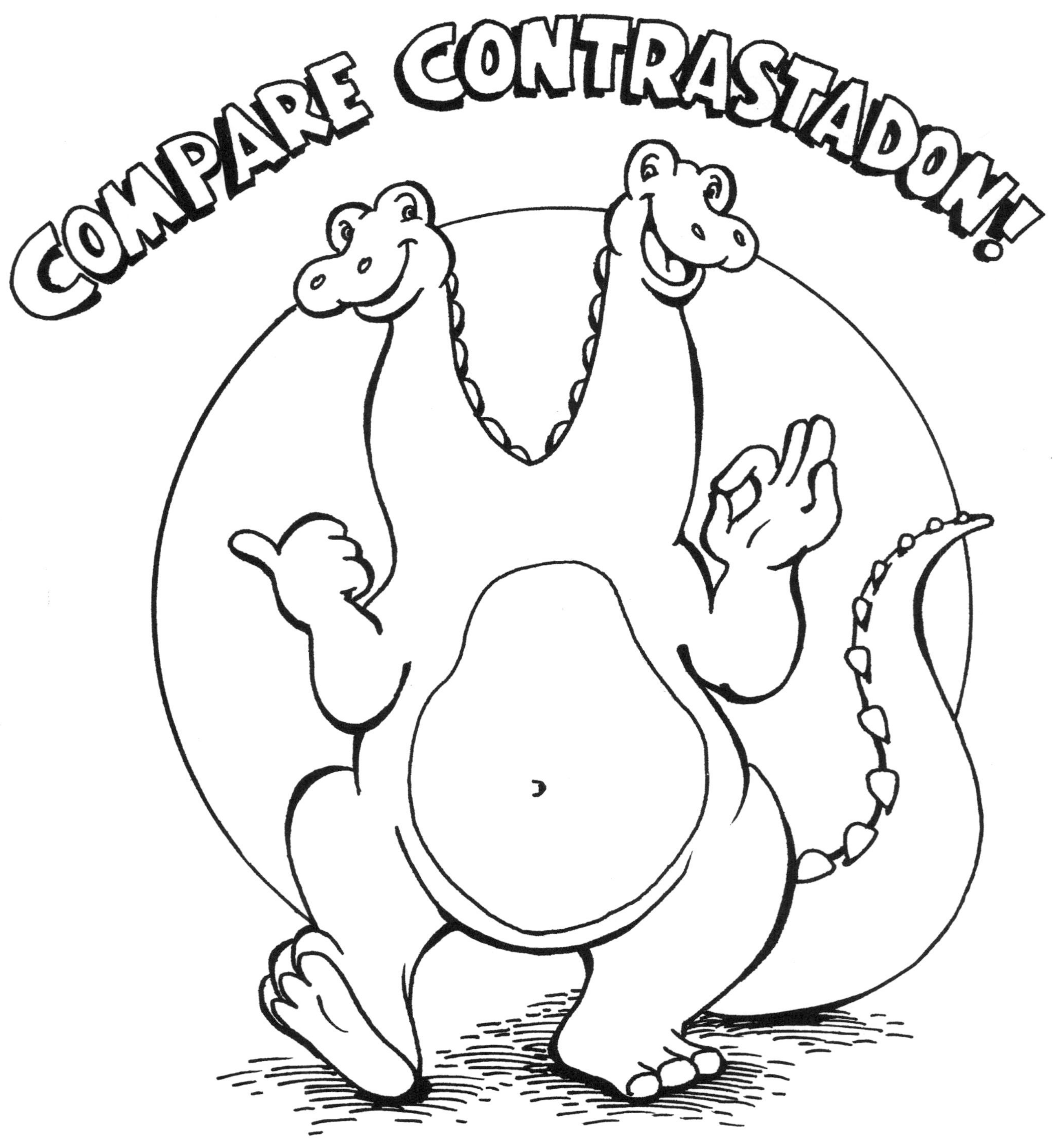
COMPARE CONTRASTADON!

LASSO THE WORD HERD and COMPARE CONTRASTADON FOLLOW-UP ACTIVITIES

GOAL

To reinforce and review *Lasso the Word Herd* and *Compare Contrastadon* strategies

BACKGROUND INFORMATION

The main focus of this lesson is to review the previous two strategies. The strategy guide review pages will be compiled with similar pages into a booklet. This booklet, along with a vacation calendar, provide a means of practicing with family members and reinforcing skills throughout a school break. Although some educators may choose to do the strategy guide pages and homework activities at the end of each lesson, others prefer delayed reinforcement to strengthen knowledge of strategies, concepts, and vocabulary covered within the lessons. Using a small representation of the strategy poster, the strategy guide pages include the specific vocabulary from the lessons. An application component is provided on the second pages of the strategy guides. Students may do reflective writing about how the strategy is or can be useful to them.

OBJECTIVES

1. Tell and write the major components of the *Lasso the Word Herd* and *Compare Contrastadon* strategies.
2. Reflect and write about how the strategies will help at home, at school, and in the community.
3. Share strategy information with family members and complete the application activities.

MATERIALS

1. *Lasso the Word Herd* poster (Created earlier)
2. *Compare Contrastadon* poster (Created earlier)
3. *Lasso the Word Herd Strategy Guide* (See pages 134–135; duplicate one per student.)
4. *Compare Contrastadon Strategy Guide* (See pages 136–137; duplicate one per student.)
5. *Lasso the Word Herd Homework Activity* (See page 138; duplicate one per student.)
6. *Compare Contrastadon Homework Activity* (See page 139; duplicate one per student.)

INTRODUCTION

Tie-in to Prior Learning

Remind the students that they have now learned two more strategies that will help them move toward achieving their goals to improve their describing skills. Display the posters and review the *Lasso the Word Herd* and *Compare Contrastadon* strategies. Have students tell about each of the strategies in their own words.

Focus/Relevancy

Review the importance of the *Strategy Guide Booklet* which will be a collection of the student's strategy guide pages for each strategy learned. The booklet will help them become better communicators by helping them remember all the strategies they will be learning. Remind students that new pages are added as new strategies are learned. Say to them,

> *We're ready to add the next pages to our* Strategy Guide Booklet *to help us remember the importance of organizing and categorizing and comparing and contrasting.*

LESSON ACTIVITIES

1. Distribute the *Lasso the Word Herd Strategy Guide Pages*. Break the large group into small groups of three or four. In the small groups, have one student be the writer and think of a category idea. Explain to the writers that they are to write two or three members of a category within the lasso on the first page of their strategy guide sheets. They may want to write the category name on the back of the page. The rest of the group will guess the category by naming other members of the group as in playing the "In Crowd—Out Crowd" game. (If necessary, list category ideas on the board for students who are having difficulty thinking of their own [e.g., pets, circus animals, zoo animals, things with stripes, things that melt, large things].) Have group members each take a turn being the writer.

2. On the second page of the strategy guide, have students write how this particular strategy has helped them or will help them at school, at home, or in the community. Brainstorm ideas (e.g., "When I clean my room, I group things that are alike in my dresser like socks in the sock drawer," "I help put groceries away and they are grouped with things that are alike in the cupboard," "In science class, we talked about animals that are mammals. I know animals that fit in that group").

3. Distribute the *Compare Contrastadon Strategy Guide* pages. Students should demonstrate they know the strategy by completing the page. Give an example of how the strategy guide can be used to organize ideas to compare and contrast. List several pairs of objects on the board that students can choose from for their strategy guide page. Tell them to choose a pair of objects and write how they are alike and different on the compare contrastadon. Refer to the poster if necessary. After writing how the two objects compare and contrast, have each student tell about their objects. Emphasize the use of specific words when telling their comparison statements. A lead-in phrase such as "The ___ and the ___ are alike because… and they are different because…" is helpful for some students.

4. On the second page of the strategy guide, have students write how each particular strategy has helped them or will help them at school, at home, or in the community. Brainstorm ideas (e.g., "I can figure out how to find a book in the library now because I know how the books are grouped," "I compare and contrast when I make decisions about how to spend my money").

5. Hand out the *Lasso the Word Herd* and the *Compare Contrastadon Homework Activity* pages and discuss them. Reinforce the importance of sharing this information with family members, and the ease and fun of doing these assignments. They will only take a few minutes to complete, but students can impress their families with what they have learned! Have a reward system established to encourage students to bring their homework activity pages back to school signed by a family member.

CLOSURE

Summarize the lesson, review its relevance to students, and tie it to future learning. Discuss the objectives that were completed in this review (i.e., the students can tell and write the *Lasso the Word Herd* and *Compare Contrastadon* strategies; they can tell how they will use the strategies; they know the strategies well enough to share them with their family members).

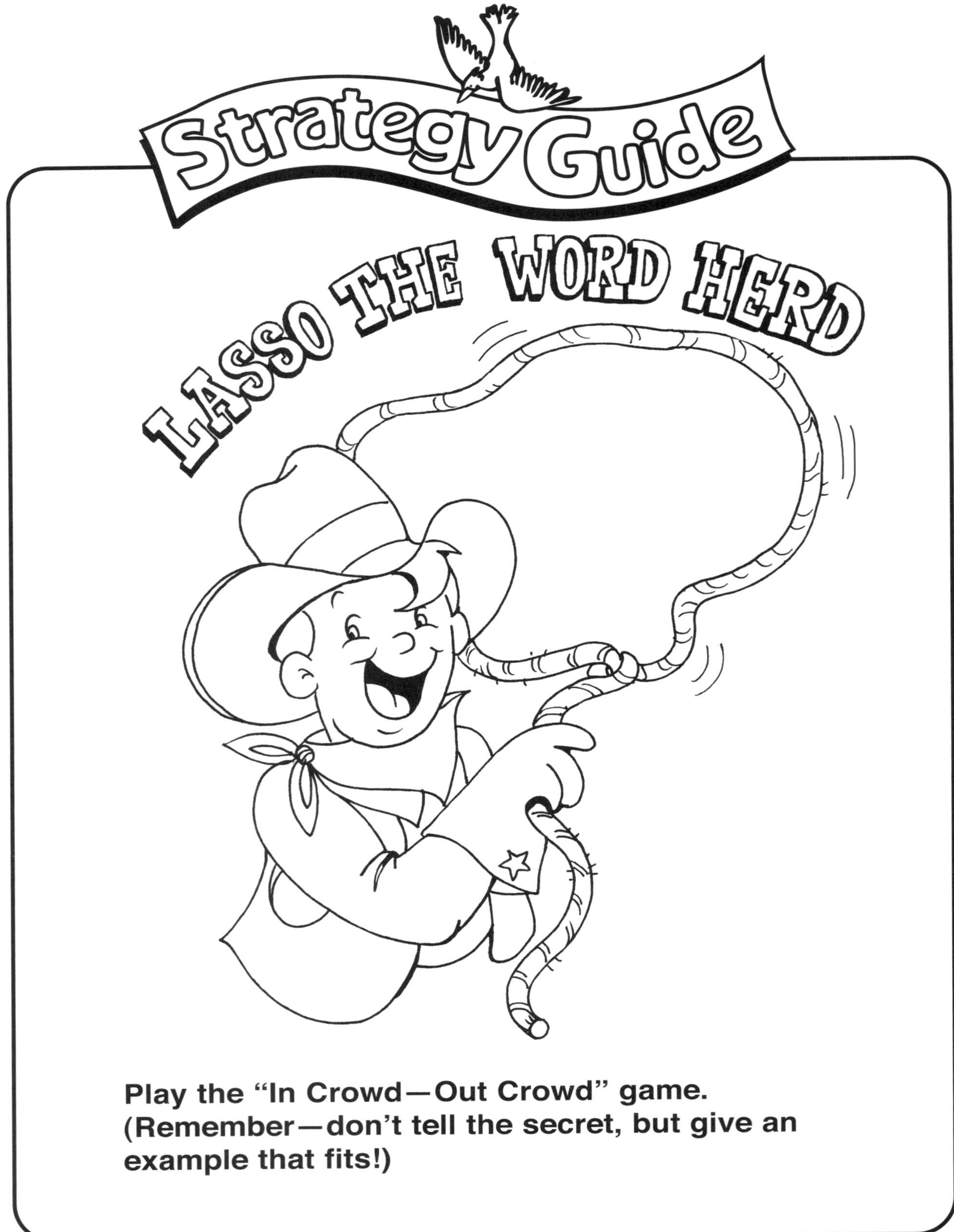

Play the "In Crowd—Out Crowd" game. (Remember—don't tell the secret, but give an example that fits!)

Lasso the Word Herd: Categorization

Name: ____________________ Date: __________

Directions: Write a sentence about how you have used or will use the strategy in each place.

At home, I ____________________

At school, I ____________________

In my community, I ____________________

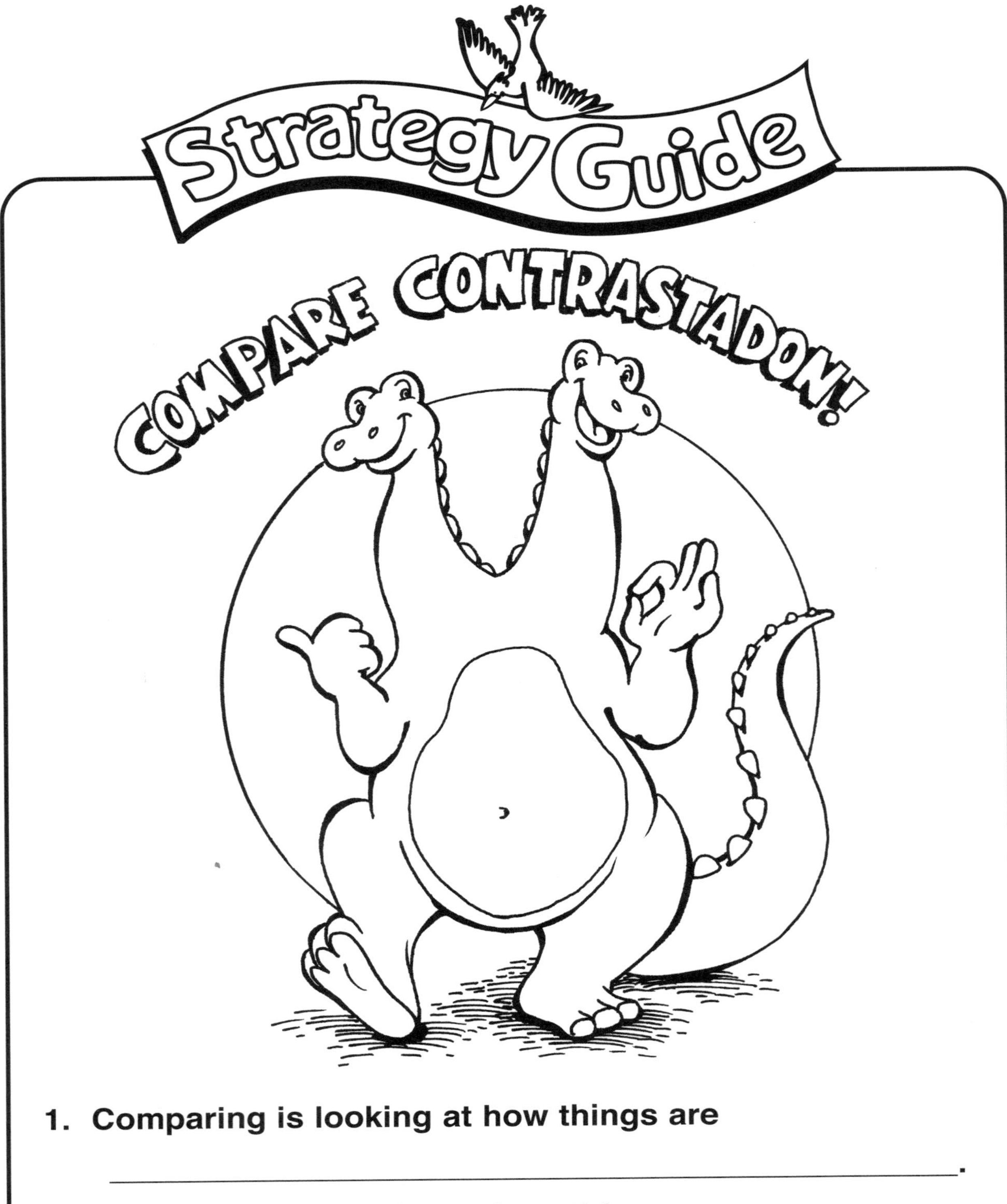

1. Comparing is looking at how things are

___________________________________.

2. Contrasting is looking at how things are

___________________________________.

Compare Contrastadon: Comparing and Contrasting

Name: ______________________________ Date: ______________

Directions: Write a sentence about how you have used or will use the strategy in each place.

At home, I ____

____

____

____

____

____

At school, I ____

____

____

____

____

____

In my community, I ____

____

____

____

____

____

Homework Activity

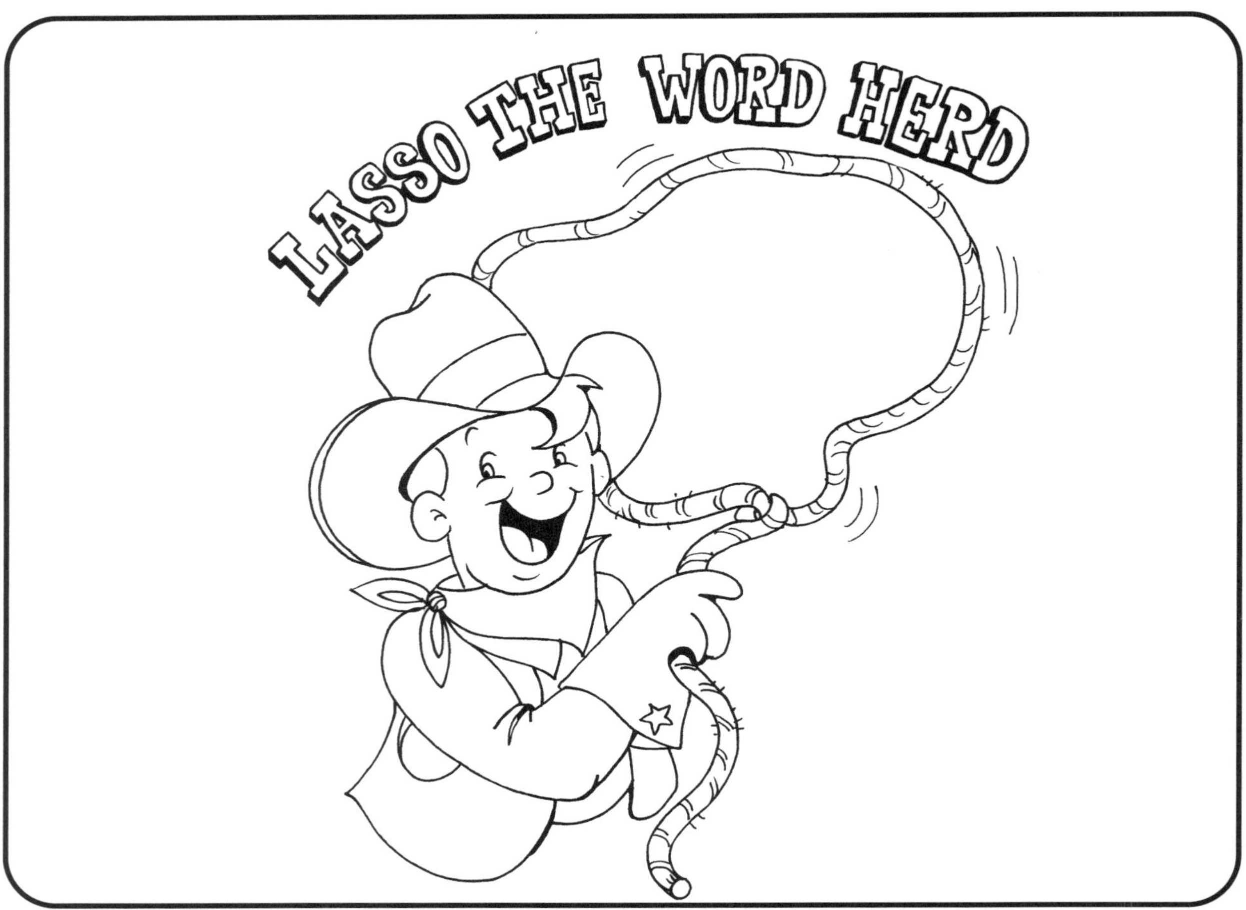

Dear Family,

1. Have your child explain the *Lasso the Word Herd* strategy and tell why it's important to know how things are categorized or organized.
2. Ask your child to name three words that go together and tell the category name (e.g., rose, tulip, and sunflower).
3. The next time you are in a grocery store together, have your child name the category of food for each aisle or area (e.g., frozen foods, produce, meat department, etc.). On the way home, name a category and ask your child to name two items that would be found there.
4. If your child completes these activities, please sign below and return this form to school.

Family Member: ______________________________ Date: ____________________

Homework Activity

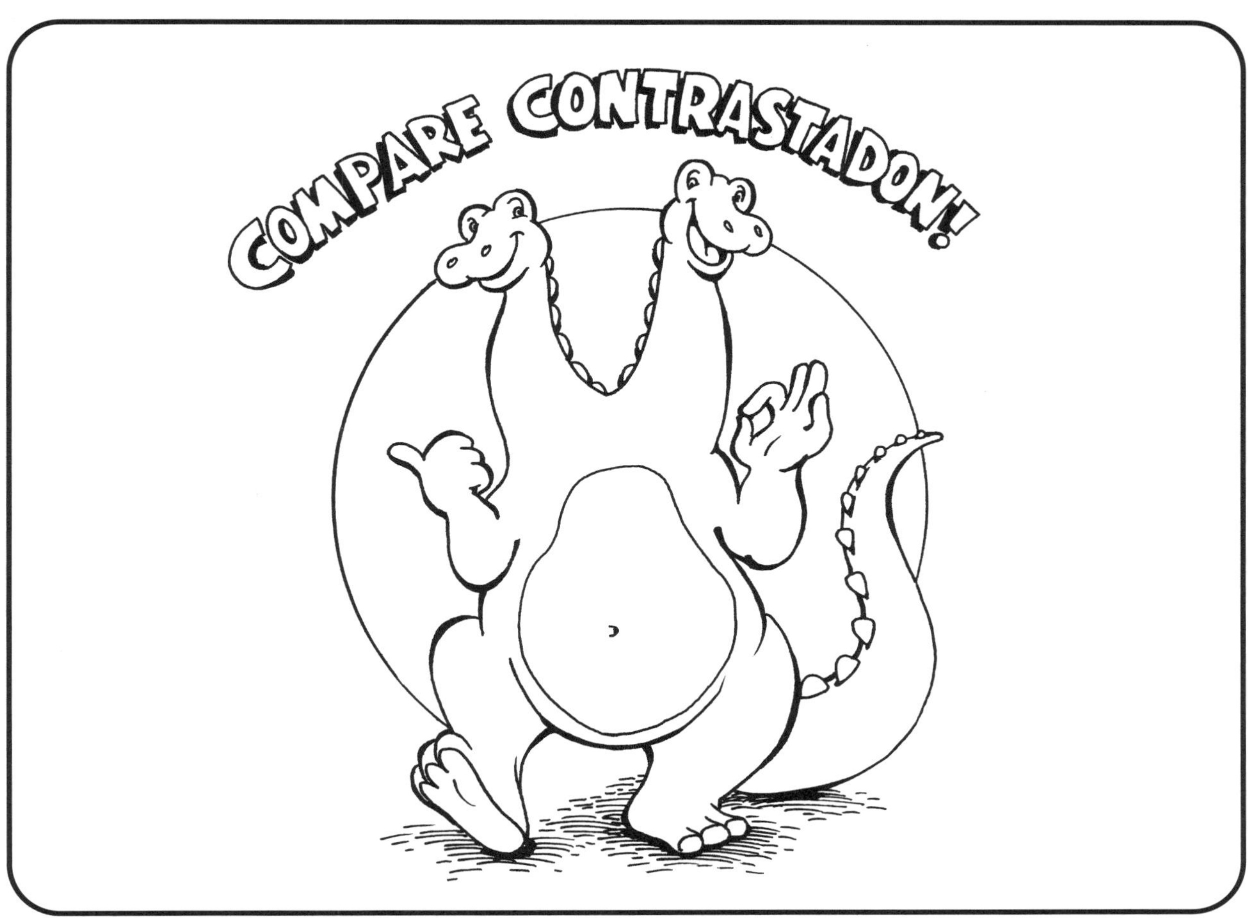

Dear Family,

1. Have your child explain the *Compare Contrastadon* strategy and tell why it's important to compare and contrast things.
2. Ask your child to compare and contrast word pairs by telling two ways the words are alike and two ways they are different. Here are some pairs:

couch—chair	desert—jungle	rain—snow
soda pop–juice	school—home	vegetables—fruit

3. If your child completes these activities, please sign below and return this form to school.

Family Member: ________________________________ Date: ______________________

GOAL SETTING ACTIVITY THREE

GOAL

To encourage self-improvement through goal setting

BACKGROUND INFORMATION

The main focus of the goal-setting lesson is to help students learn the steps for goal setting (i.e., identifying a need, formulating a goal, practicing the steps to reach the goal, revising a goal as needed, and evaluating progress toward meeting a goal). Rather than expecting students to set goals independently, the goal-setting process is modeled. The communication goal could be directed by you, but the reflection on how the goal might be useful will be individual for each student, since each student's use of the skills will be different. A few example goals for this unit are:

1. Improve word power;
2. Use word power to solve problems; and
3. Use precise and clear definitions.

OBJECTIVES

1. Evaluate progress on achieving previously set goals.
2. Tell how previous goals were met.
3. Write a new goal.

MATERIALS

1. *My Goals #3* (See page 142; duplicate one per student.)
2. *My Goals #2* (Completed in *Goal Setting Activity Two*)
3. Chalkboard and chalk

INTRODUCTION

Tie-in to Prior Learning

Remind students that in *Goal Setting Activity Two* they had identified specific skills that would strengthen their communication, especially categorizing, and comparing and contrasting.

Focus/Relevancy

1. Explain to students that they will be evaluating their progress on achieving previous goals set and will write new goals to achieve.

2. Remind students that learning is easier when goals are set and there is a plan for practicing. Setting goals can help students achieve many different skills, both in school and at home. Discuss how it feels to accomplish something that was difficult.

LESSON ACTIVITIES

1. Give each student a copy of *My Goals #3* and their completed *My Goals #2*. Review the words *achieve, revise,* and *repeat*. Review the strategies and vocabulary learned. Have students evaluate ways that their categorization and comparing and contrasting skills have improved and ask them to give examples (e.g., "I know how the library categorizes books, so now it's easier for me to find what I'm looking for," "I can help my dad find food in the grocery store because I know how the groceries are grouped in the aisles," "I compare and contrast before I make choices"). Ask students to complete the first half of *My Goals #3*. Have them check whether they achieved their goals or whether they need to revise their goals. Remind students that they will want to continue to practice each achieved goal while targeting another for improvement.

2. Point out the "My new goal is" sentence on the goal sheet. To prompt the discussion of a new goal, ask students if they ever have a problem knowing what a word means or thinking of the right word to say. Tell them that the next strategies they learn will help them improve their "word power." Write the words *word power* on the board and ask the students for predictions of what *word power* means. As the students share ideas, relate to them the targeted skills of understanding and using synonyms, antonyms, and multiple meaning words; defining words clearly; and using words to solve analogies. If the students express that *word power* means "knowing lots of words," validate this response by sharing how having word power helps them be better communicators. Develop the concept that word power enables students to play with language in many exciting ways (e.g., to understand analogies, to tell and understand jokes and riddles, etc.).

3. Write goals such as, *Improve word power,* or *Use word power to solve problems,* on the board for students to add to their goal sheets.

CLOSURE

Summarize the lesson, review its relevance for students, and tie it to future learning. Remind students that they have set important goals. And remind students that by signing and dating their goal sheets, they are promising to concentrate and work on their goals. On the bottom of the goal sheets is a line for a family member's signature. Have students take the goal sheets home, explain their goals to their family members, and return the goal sheets to school for you to sign.

My Goals #3

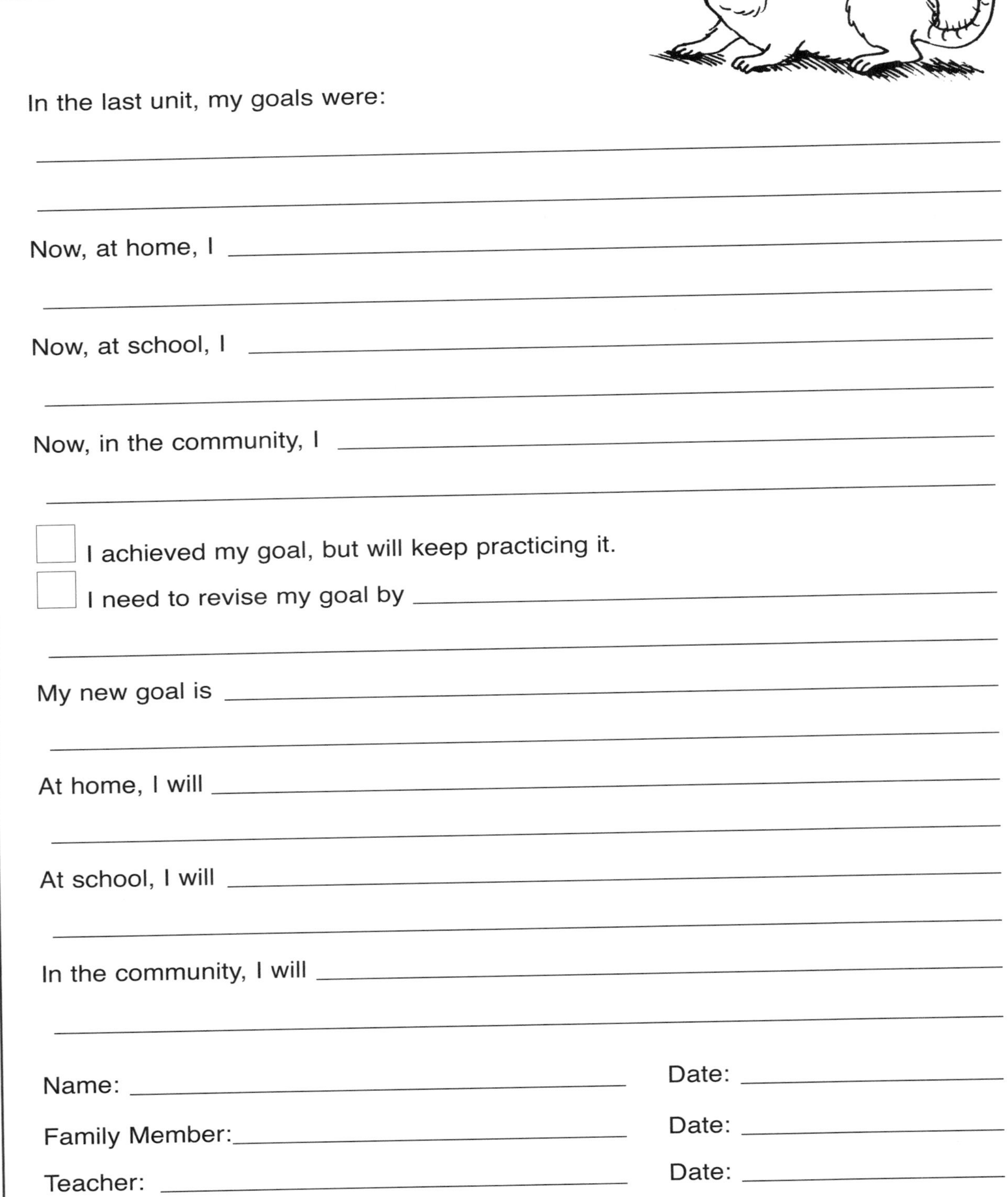

In the last unit, my goals were:

____

____

Now, at home, I ______________________________

____

Now, at school, I _____________________________

____

Now, in the community, I _______________________

____

☐ I achieved my goal, but will keep practicing it.

☐ I need to revise my goal by ____________________

____

My new goal is ________________________________

____

At home, I will _______________________________

____

At school, I will ______________________________

____

In the community, I will ________________________

____

Name: ____________________ Date: __________

Family Member: ______________ Date: __________

Teacher: ___________________ Date: __________

WEIGH THE MEANING: SYNONYMS AND ANTONYMS

GOAL

To develop vocabulary skills

BACKGROUND INFORMATION

The *Weigh the Meaning* strategy is part of a series of strategies to develop the students' expressive and receptive vocabulary knowledge. The lessons work to build flexibility of word knowledge and use. These lessons are presented to the students as a way to develop their "word power" so that they can be more creative in their understanding and usage of language.

The concept of knowing and using synonyms is presented using a self-prompting question and the concept of knowing and using antonyms is presented using a cloze technique. The self-prompting question strategy for synonyms uses the idea of "balancing" the meaning using a graphic of a scale. Students ask themselves: Does the meaning stay the same in the sentence? The cloze technique for prompting a one-word antonym is the sentence "It's not _____, but _____." The students think not _____, then give the one-word opposite.

In this lesson, there is reference to the book *This Is My House,* which was read in the *Compare Contrastadon* lesson. If a different book was read in that lesson, the *Focus/Relevancy* of this lesson will need to be adapted.

OBJECTIVES

1. Understand and use synonyms and use them appropriately in sentences.
2. Generate a one-word antonym when given a word.

MATERIALS

1. Chalkboard and chalk
2. *Climate Chart* (See page 147; create one transparency.)
3. Overhead projector
4. Water soluble marker
5. *Weigh the Meaning* graphic (See page 148; duplicate and enlarge the graphic, color it, mount it onto poster board, and laminate it for durability, if desired.)
6. Thesaurus (One per small group of three or four students)
7. *Antonym Word Lists (Levels I, II, III)* (See pages 149–151; duplicate one per small group of students.)

INTRODUCTION

Tie-in to Prior Learning

Discuss with students that using the *Lasso the Word Herd* strategy, they were organizing and grouping words together that were alike in some way. Elicit the concept of categorization. Remind students that they also used the *Compare Contrastadon* strategy to help organize ideas by comparing their similarities and contrasting the differences. Review these two strategies if necessary. Remind students that these strategies will help them strengthen their word power but there are several other strategies they will learn that are powerful word tools.

Focus/Relevancy

1. Discuss what the word *power* means. Elicit different meanings, such as *energy, control,* and *strength*. Say to the students,

   We can be more powerful communicators through the words we choose when expressing our ideas.

2. Remind students about how descriptive and informative their sentences were when they used their senses to describe (i.e., using the *It Makes Sense* strategy) and stress that they will be learning two other ways to make their ideas clear and more vivid for the listener or reader. They will be learning about the power of synonyms and antonyms. Ask the students if they have heard of these words before. Have students brainstorm what they think these words mean and write their responses on the board.

3. Remind students that the story *This Is My House* told about people's homes around the world. Discuss the climate (i.e., weather, temperature) factors that might influence the type of home that is built in a particular region. Display the *Climate Chart* overhead transparency. Choose two contrasting regions to highlight (e.g., mountain region and the desert). Have the students brainstorm words to describe the regions, such as *cold, rugged, snow-capped peaks* for the mountain region; *hot, sandy, cactus* for the desert region. Write the words in the appropriate space on the *Climate Chart*. Explain that students will use these words to learn a strategy that will build word power.

4. Write several sentences on the board or chart using the information from the desert region (e.g., "When I visited the desert, the sand was hot. The wind was hot on my face. The cactus stood in the hot sun"). Have students evaluate the sentences. Elicit the idea of redundancy of the word *hot* and the need for word power to make the sentences more interesting to the listener or reader. Tell students that learning about synonyms and antonyms will help to make their speaking and writing more interesting and entertaining.

LESSON ACTIVITIES

1. Show the *Weigh the Meaning* poster. Discuss what a balancing scale is. Tell students that in this lesson a scale is used to compare word meanings. Draw a similar scale on the board. Write the word *hot* on one side of the scale. Refer back to the desert sentences written on the board or on the transparency. Say to the students,

   We wrote that "The sand was hot, the wind was hot, the sun was hot." To give our sentences more power we could use synonyms, or words that have the same meaning. (Write the word *synonym* on the board and have students use whisper voices [see page 13] to say *synonym.) Synonyms can make sentences more interesting without changing the meaning.*

2. Have a student generate a word that would have the same meaning as *hot* (e.g., *blazing, fiery, broiling*) and write it on the other side of the scale. Point out the balance between the two words (e.g., The sentences, "The sand was hot" and "The sand was blazing," would weigh the same on the scale). Repeat this process with the other two synonyms. To decide if two words are synonyms, students can ask themselves, "Does the meaning stay the same in the sentence?"

3. For additional practice generating synonyms, show students how a thesaurus can help them find synonyms. Break students into small groups of three or four. Give each group a thesaurus. Write several words on the board (one for each group) and have groups look up the particular word in the thesaurus. Example words are: *cold, hot, fast, large, happy, excite, sad*. Have one spokesperson from each group read some of the synonym choices. Stress the similarities in meaning of the synonyms for each word, and how these synonyms could make interesting and powerful communication.

4. Write the words *hot* and *warm* on each side of the scale. Discuss how to position the scale to show a slight imbalance using a sentence context (e.g., "I walked on the hot sand" or "I walked on the warm sand"). Have the students visualize the difference between walking on sand which is hot as compared to warm sand. These two words may be in the same family, but they do not exactly balance the scale. Have one student redraw the scale to show the imbalance. Refer students to the poster and remind them that synonyms will weigh the same and won't change the meaning of a sentence.

5. Explain to students that another important skill for speaking and writing in interesting and entertaining ways is to use antonyms. Ask students what they think an antonym is and write their responses on the board. Discuss the meaning of antonym by reminding students that antonyms are opposites. Draw two ants on the board going in opposite directions (e.g., one

going left and one right) to illustrate the meaning. Have students use whisper voices (see page 13) to say the word *antonym*.

6. Show the *Weigh the Meaning* poster and point out the cave characters Ig and Ug. Say to the students,

   This is Ig and Ug who will help us think about antonyms. Ug isn't a very efficient language user. He has to use more words to get his message across. When he holds his hands to the fire, he thinks, "Not cold." Ig is a much better communicator. She thinks, "Hot." She gets her message across quickly and precisely, using one word. Point out the phrase that is part of the graphic, "Not cold but hot." We're going to practice using this phrase to give the opposites of words.

7. Divide the students into small groups. Appoint a spokesperson for each group. Let the group choose to complete a *Level I* (easiest), *Level II* (harder), or *Level III* (hardest) *Antonym Word List* activity page. Have each group confer together to complete the page. Remind them to think of the phrase, "Not _____, but _____." At the end of the time period, check to see if any group had a sentence they could not solve and, if so, to present it to the larger group to solve. Then have each small group ask the larger group to solve the antonym sentence that they created.

CLOSURE

Summarize the lesson, review its relevance to students, and tie it to future learning. Tell the students that they are now experts at thinking of antonyms and synonyms. Remind students of the resource they can use to find synonyms of words. Highlight the fact that since the students have worked on antonyms, synonyms, categorization, and description, they are now prepared to use their new word power to solve analogies.

Climate Chart

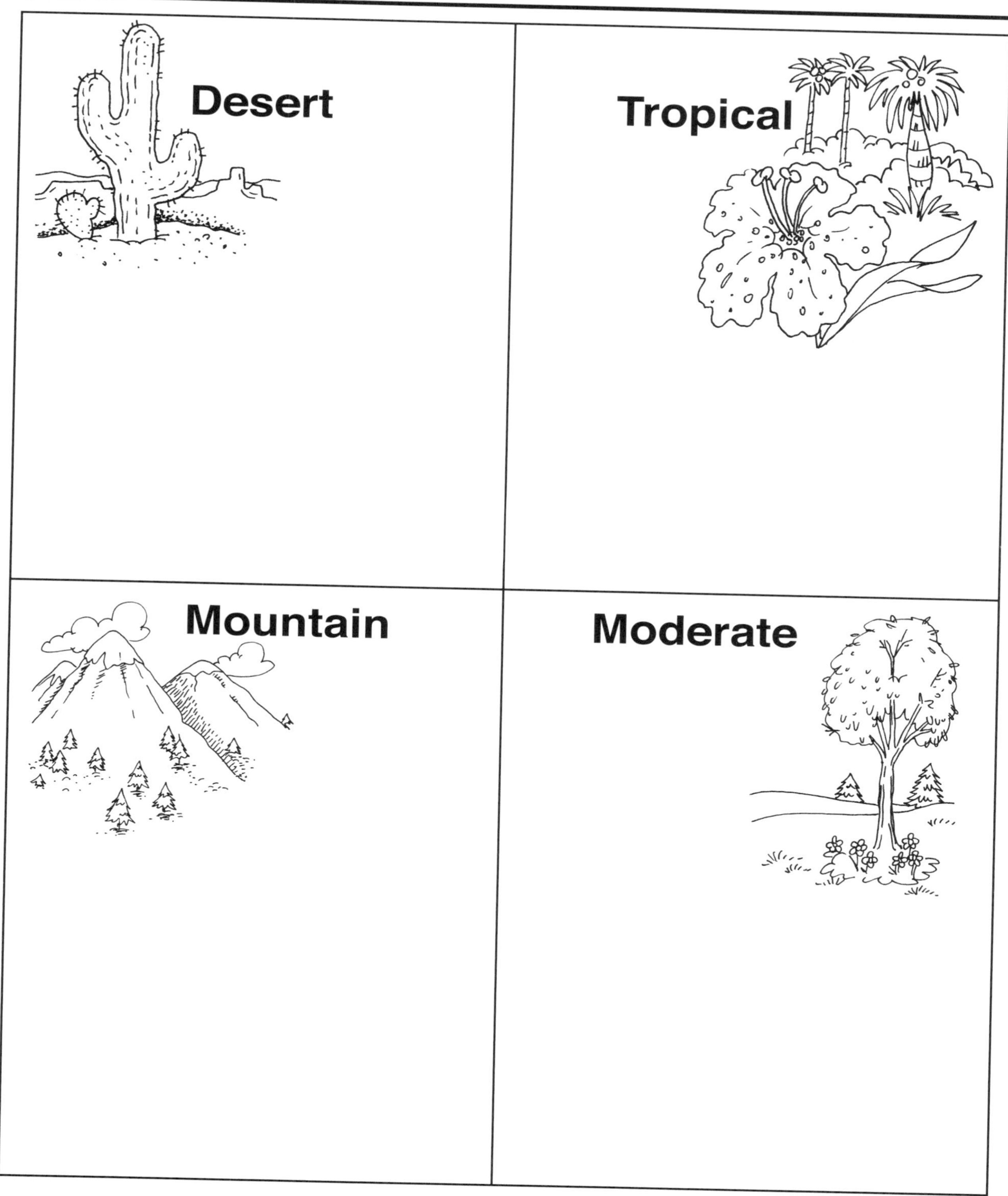

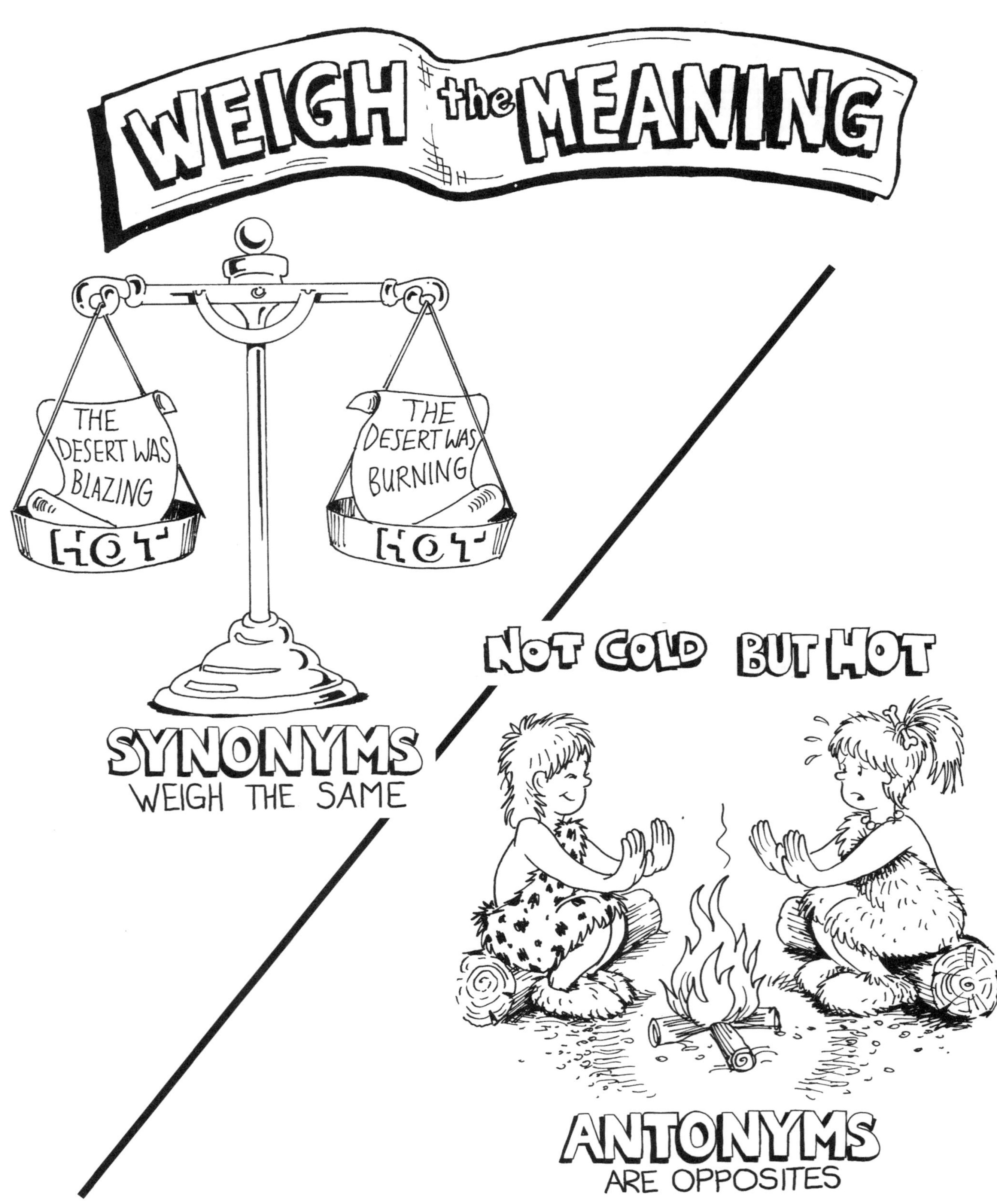
WEIGH the MEANING
THE DESERT WAS BLAZING
THE DESERT WAS BURNING
HOT
HOT
SYNONYMS
WEIGH THE SAME
NOT COLD BUT HOT
ANTONYMS
ARE OPPOSITES

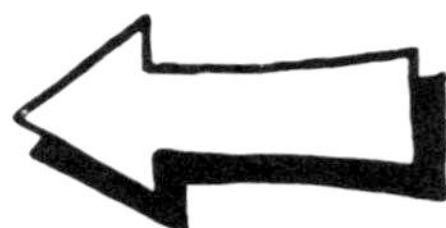

Antonym Word List Level I

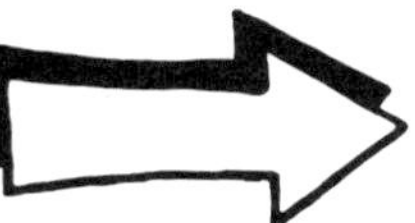

Name: ______________________ Date: __________

Directions: Complete the sentences by writing a word that is opposite on the blank lines.

1. It's not morning, it's ______________________.
2. We're not in the city, we're in the ______________________.
3. She's not laughing, she's ______________________.
4. The box isn't heavy, it's ______________________.
5. The party is not quiet, it's ______________________.
6. The dog is not in the doghouse, it's ______________________.
7. The glass is not empty, it's ______________________.
8. The math assignment is not easy, it's ______________________.
9. It's not time to play, it's time to ______________________.
10. The towel is not dry, it's ______________________.

Create your own antonym sentences:

____

____

____

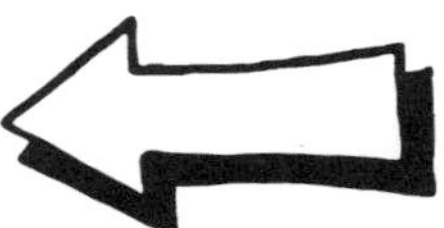

Antonym Word List Level II

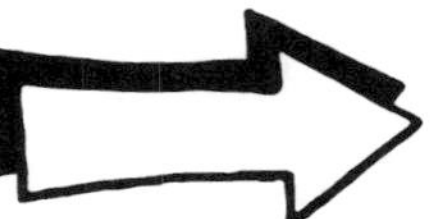

Name: ______________________________ Date: ______________

Directions: Complete the sentences by writing a word that is opposite on the blank lines.

1. The shirt is not the same, it's ______________________________.
2. The book is not an urban setting, it's ______________________________.
3. I do not want to buy a car, I want to ______________________________.
4. The paper is not wide, it's ______________________________.
5. He did not drive east, he drove ______________________________.
6. The water is not warm, it's ______________________________.
7. The jeans are not tight, they are ______________________________.
8. The knife is not dull, it's ______________________________.
9. This is not the beginning of the movie, it's the ______________________________.
10. I did not forget my money, I ______________________________.

Create your own antonym sentences:

____

____

____

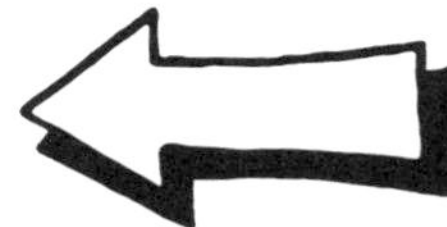

Antonym Word List Level III

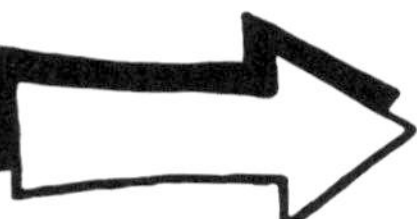

Name: ______________________ Date: __________

Directions: Complete the sentences by writing a word that is opposite on the blank lines.

1. I'm not a producer, I'm a ______________________.
2. He didn't discourage me, he ______________________.
3. The boat trip isn't dangerous, it's ______________________.
4. The experience wasn't positive, it was ______________________.
5. The paint isn't for the interior, it's for the ______________________.
6. The tool isn't useful, it's ______________________.
7. I didn't refuse the offer, I ______________________.
8. The character isn't real, it's ______________________.
9. The land isn't private, it's ______________________.
10. I'm not going to fail, I'm going to ______________________.

Create your own antonym sentences:

____

____

____

DISCOVER THE PATTERN: ANALOGIES

GOAL

To improve expressive language skills by solving analogies

BACKGROUND INFORMATION

The *Discover the Pattern* strategy has students apply what they know about vocabulary words, their word power, to solve analogies. Solving the analogies requires knowledge of vocabulary and flexibility in using the words they know. This strategy also relies on students' knowledge of categorization to recognize relationships in the analogies.

OBJECTIVES

1. Identify the pattern in an analogy.
2. Solve an analogy using words.

MATERIALS

1. Chalkboard and chalk
2. *Discover the Pattern* graphic (See page 155; duplicate and enlarge the graphic, color it, mount it onto poster board, and laminate it for durability, if desired.)
3. *Graphic Flap* (See page 156; duplicate, enlarge, and follow directions described in step 1 of *Focus/Relevancy*.)
4. Adhesive Velcro strips
5. *Analogy Relationships* (See pages 157–162; duplicate onto heavy stock paper to form posters.)
6. *Analogy Cards* (See pages 163–170; duplicate onto heavy stock paper and cut apart to form cards.)

INTRODUCTION

Tie-in to Prior Learning

Remind students that they have been studying strategies for categorizing, for comparing and contrasting ideas, and for knowing and using synonyms and antonyms. Now they are ready to apply these strategies to solve analogies.

Focus/Relevancy

1. After creating the *Discover the Pattern* poster, enlarge, duplicate, and cut out the *Graphic Flap*. The flap needs to be large enough (and not too large) to cover the first portion of the analogy as illustrated. Attach the flap to the poster using adhesive strips of Velcro.

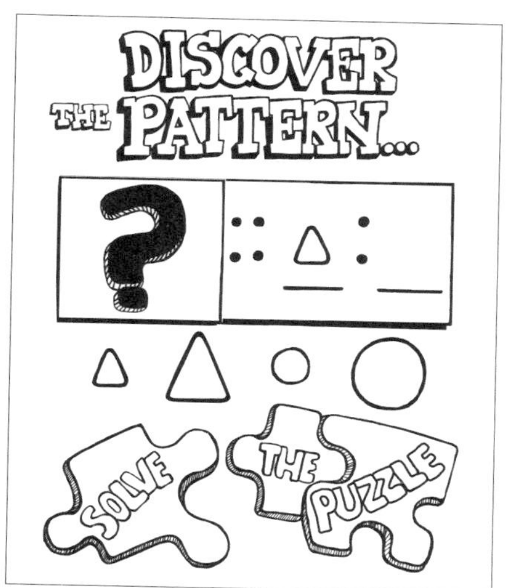

2. Introduce this strategy by writing the word *analogy* on the board and saying to the students,

   An analogy is a comparison between two things. To solve an analogy puzzle, you have to compare the two things and figure out how they are similar. The similarity creates a pattern. Who can tell me what a pattern is? (Have students give examples of various kinds of patterns.) *To be a pattern the information must be repeated in the same way each time. Recognizing the pattern or the similarity is a useful tool when working to solve analogies. The key to solving the analogy is to first discover what the pattern is.*

3. Show the *Discover the Pattern* poster. Ask if anyone can complete the analogy. Point out that possible answers are given on the poster. Students often raise their hands confidently to "solve" the puzzle. Allow students to make several guesses, then ask if anyone knows for sure what the correct answer is without seeing the pattern. Remove the *Graphic Flap* to show the rest of the pattern. Tell them that in this lesson they will be learning how to discover the pattern to solve the analogy.

LESSON ACTIVITIES

1. The analogies in this lesson are based on relationships: synonym, antonym, member/category, item/characteristic, part/whole, item/function, and item/location. These relationships are illustrated on the *Analogy Relationships* posters. Write these relationships on the board. Tell students that there are other possible patterns, but these are some of the basic patterns they will discover in this lesson. Read the relationship from the *Analogy Relationships* posters before showing them to the students. As you read from each poster, ask students to choose from the list

on the board, the relationship that applies. Allow time for students to respond to each relationship read and then display the poster that illustrates the relationship. Keep these posters visible throughout this activity. Point out that there may be more than one right answer when identifying the pattern relationships and when solving the analogies.

HINT

An extension of this activity would be to have students give an analogy that follows the same pattern.

2. Explain that the students have identified the patterns on the analogy relationship posters. Explain that analogies are written in a special way using dots to mean certain words. Show the *Discover the Pattern* poster and model how the symbols ":" and "::" are read. Say to the students,

   ":" means "is to" and "::" means "as" or "in the same way." When you read an analogy you substitute the words for the symbols. Our analogy puzzle cards will use these symbols but you will know to substitute the words in your mind when you read the analogy.

3. Explain that students will be applying this strategy to solving more analogies. Shuffle the *Analogy Cards* and deal out all cards to the students in the group. There are 63 cards, 9 of each relationship (i.e., synonym, antonym, member/category, item/characteristic, part/whole, item/function, and item/location). Notice that there is one blank card provided which may be duplicated to create your own analogies that reinforce classroom concepts or may be used to have students create analogies for others to solve.

4. Explain the procedure to students and then model the activity. Have a student read the words on one of his or her cards and identify the pattern relationship. Once the student has identified the pattern, have the other students look at their cards to see if their word pairs would finish the analogy (i.e., are the same relationship). Have at least one student complete the analogy by reading the word pairs. Continue until all the analogies have been solved. As an option, students could write the analogy responses on their cards.

CLOSURE

Summarize the lesson, review its relevance to students, and tie it to future learning. Remind the students that if they recognize the pattern, they can solve the analogy.

DISCOVER THE PATTERN...

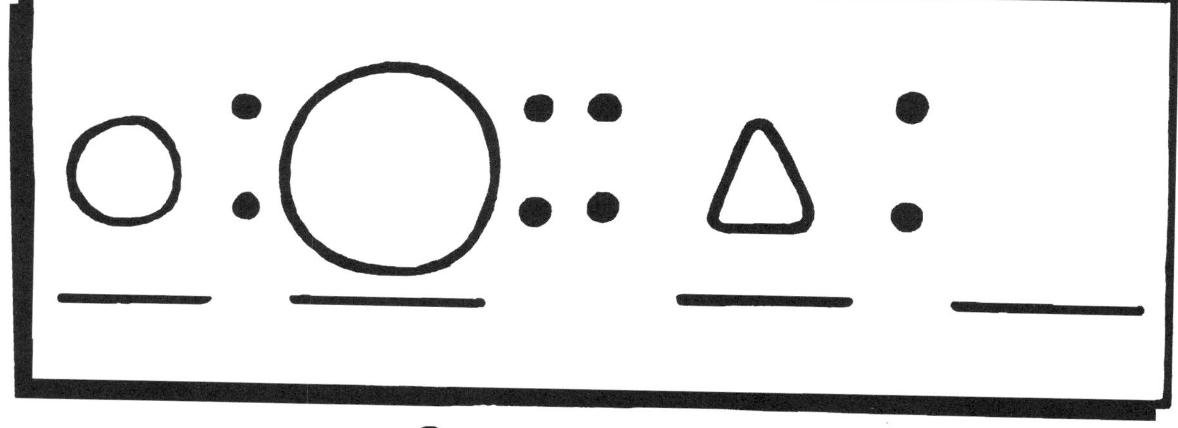

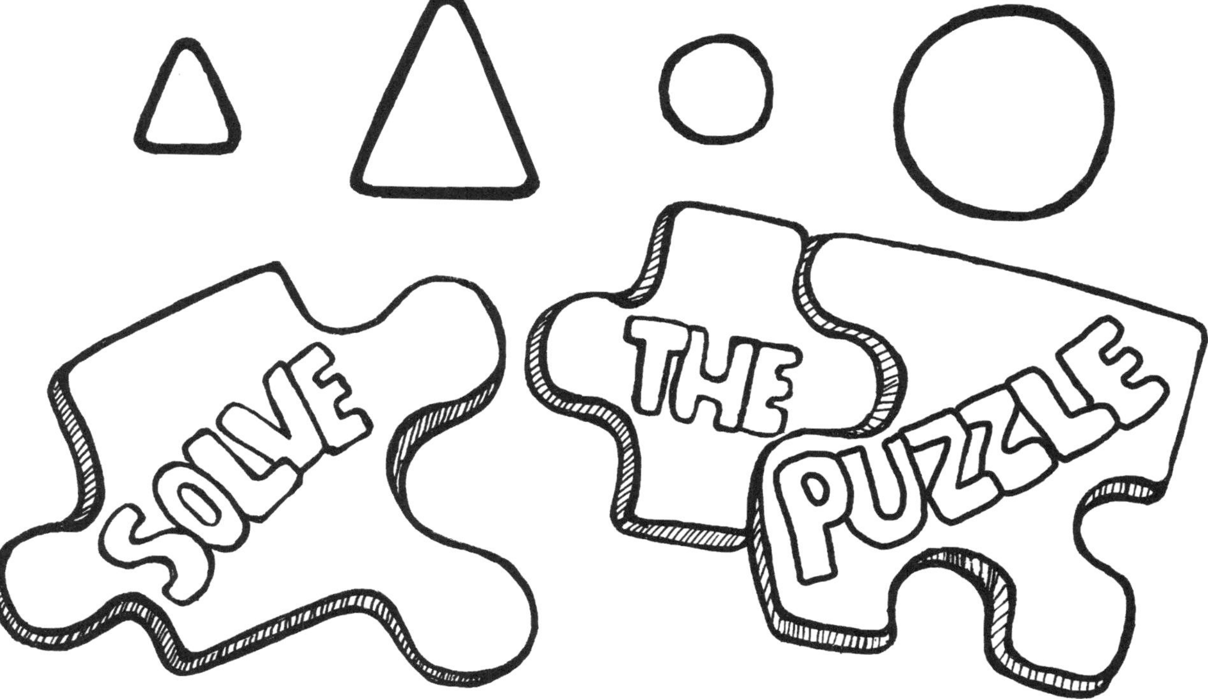

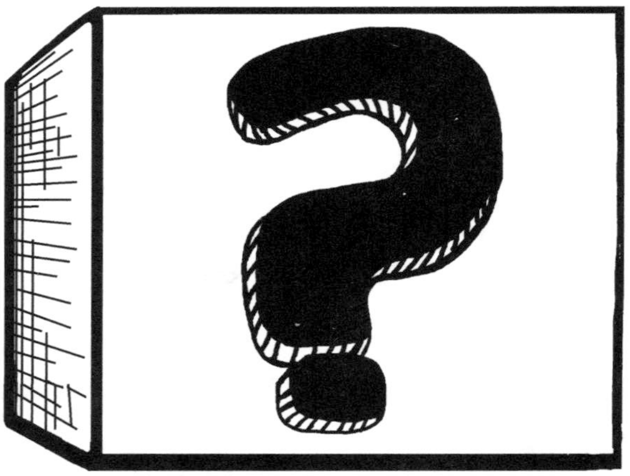

Analogy Relationships

SYNONYMS

WEIGH THE SAME

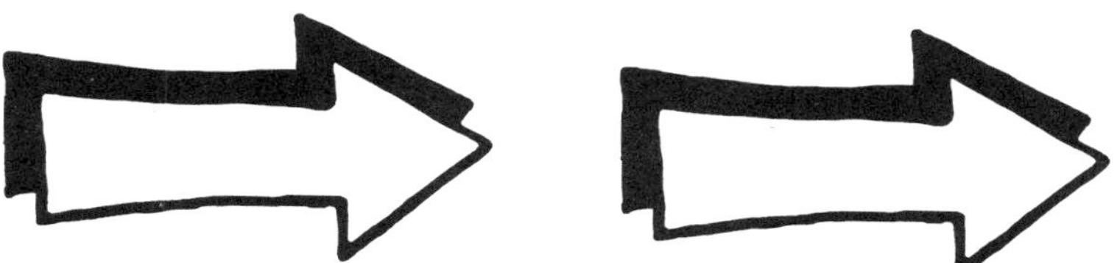

big : huge

smell : aroma

ANTONYMS

ARE OPPOSITES

rude : polite

calm : excited

Member/Category

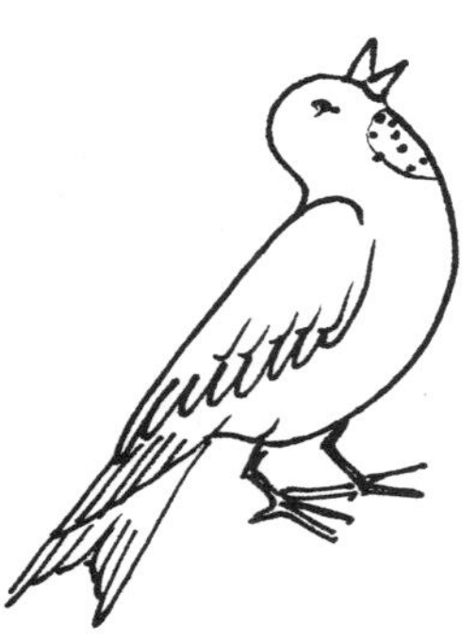

:

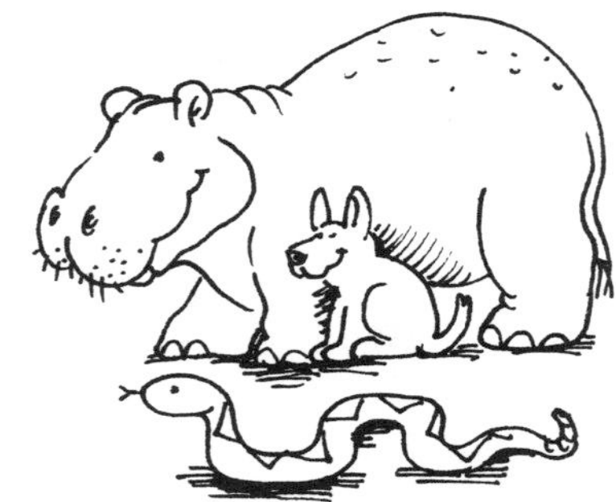

bird animals

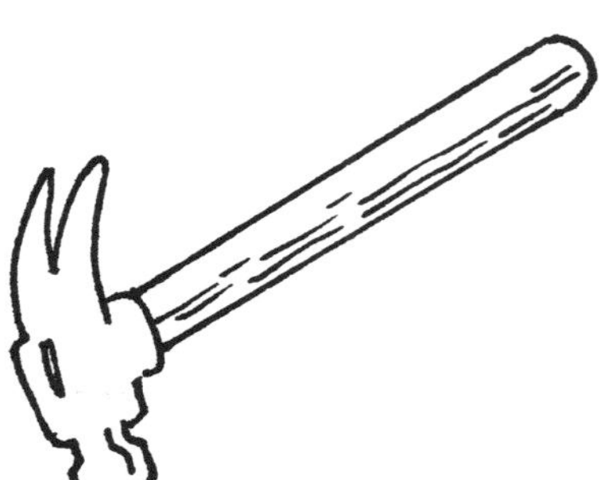

:

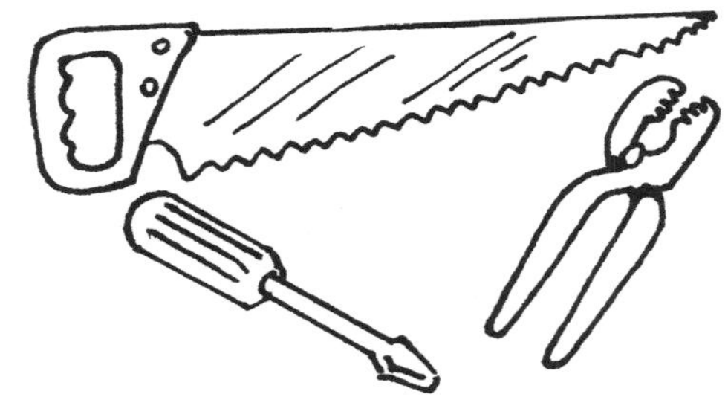

hammer tools

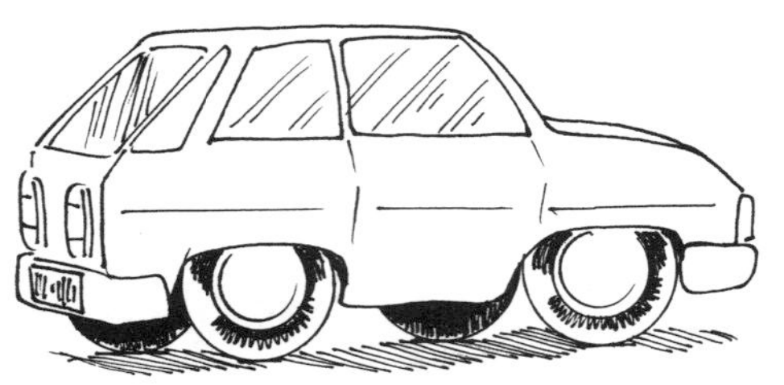

:

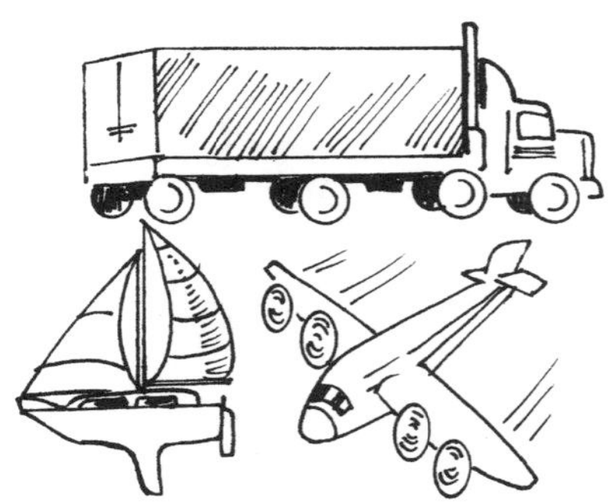

car vehicles

Item/Characteristic

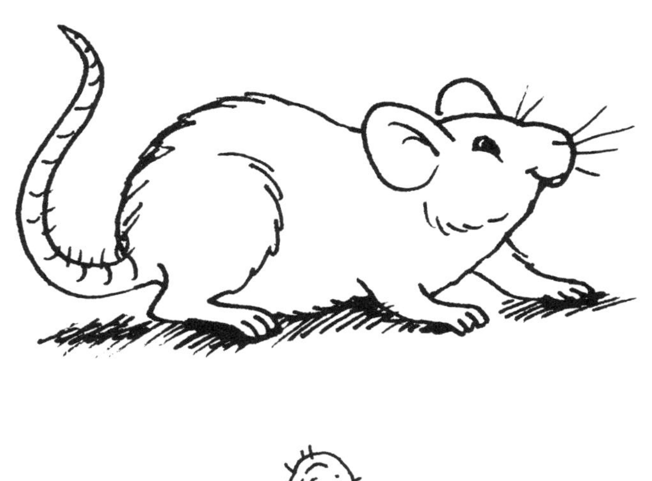

: small

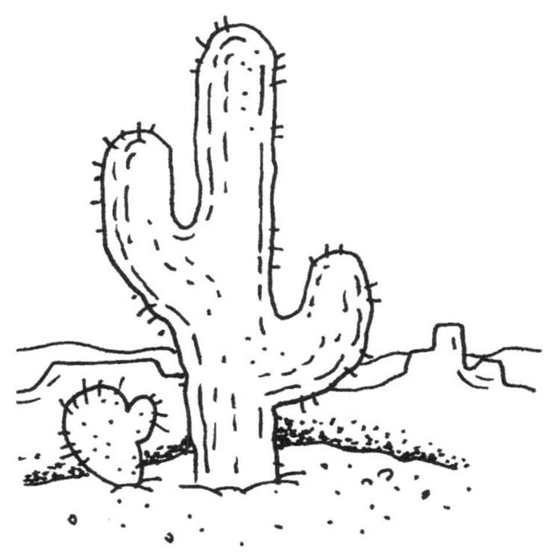

: prickly

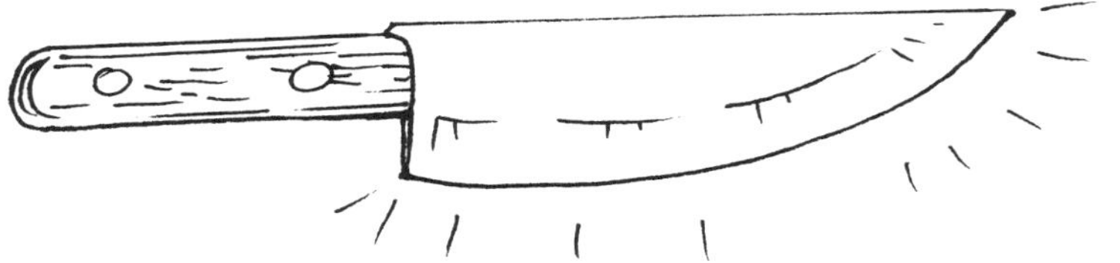

: sharp

Part/Whole

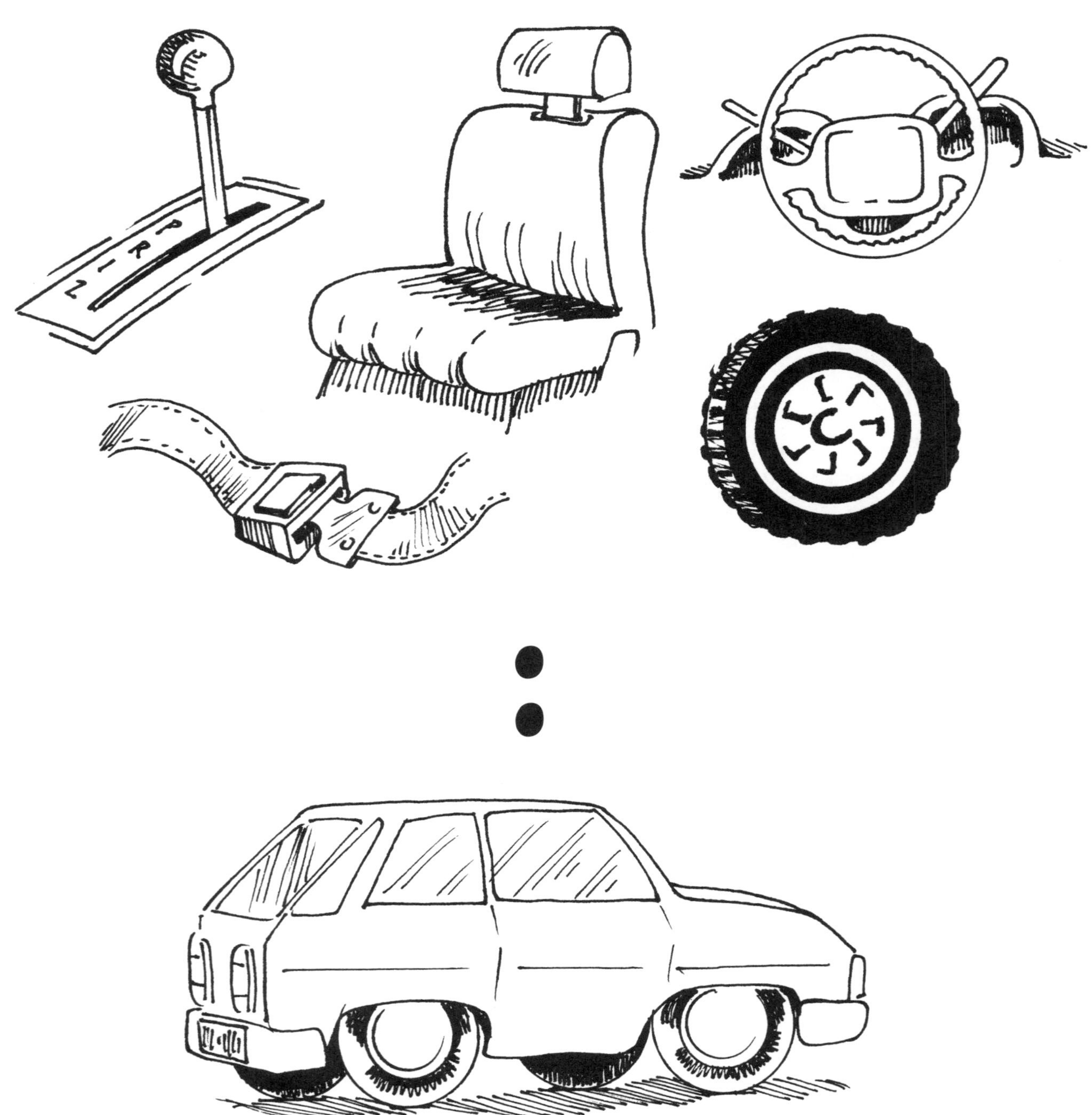

Item/Function

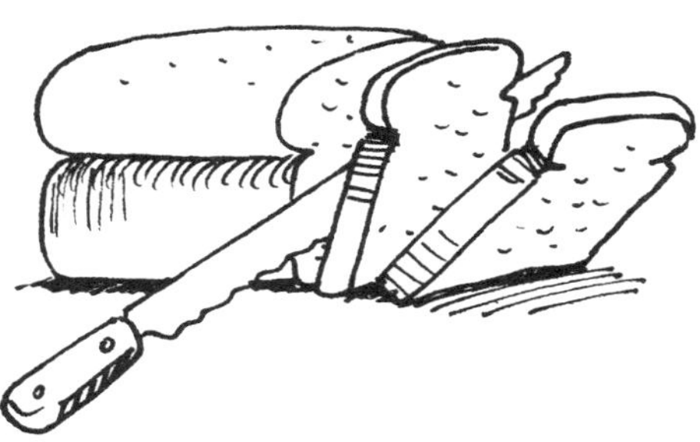

knife : cuts

pencil : writes

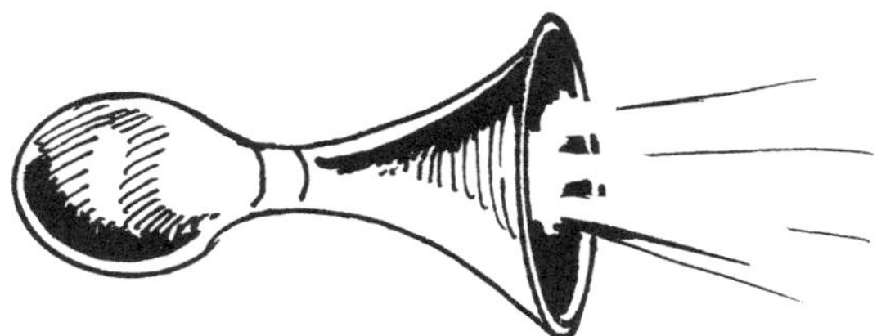

horn : honks

Item/Location

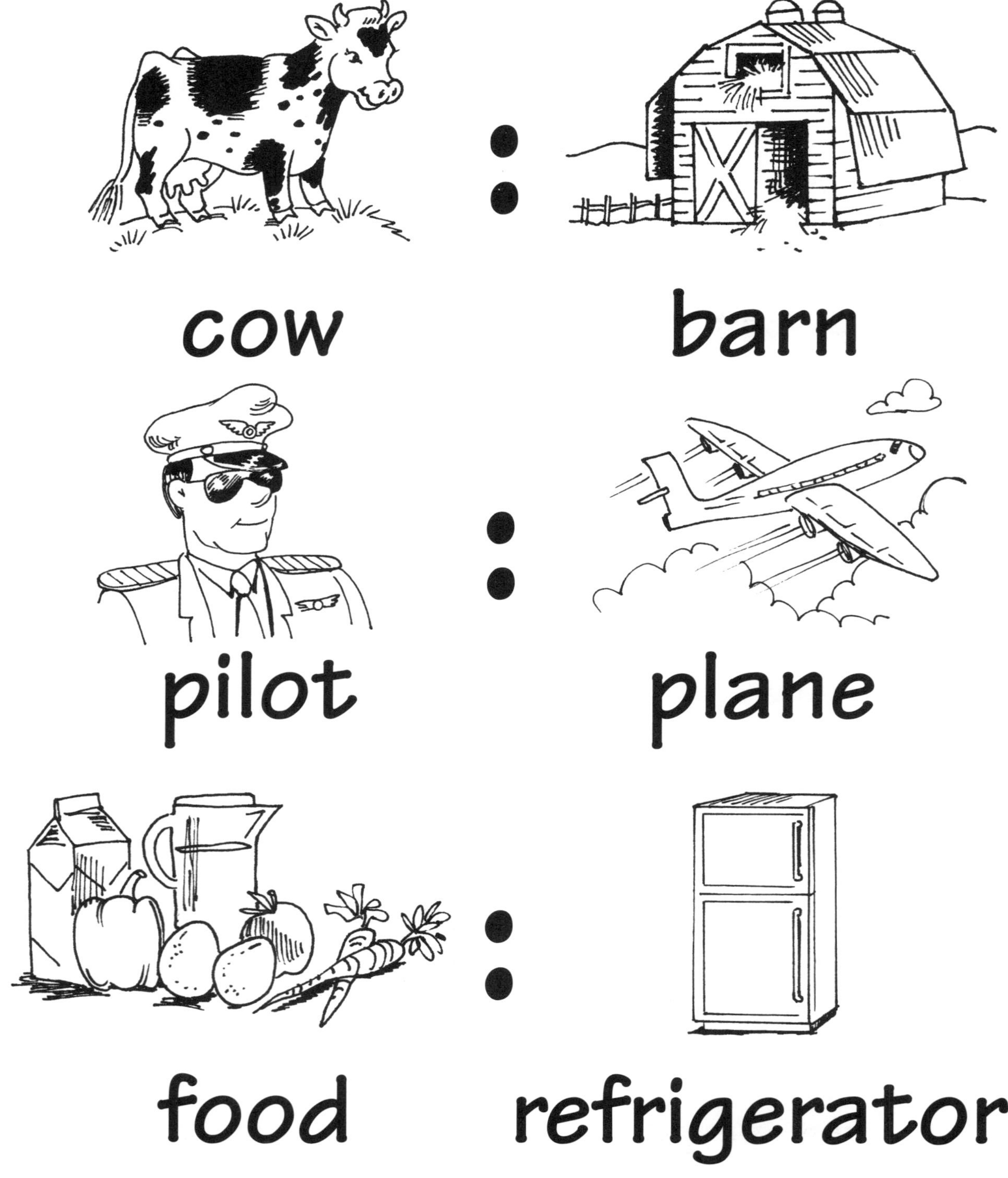

apple : red
::
_______ : _______

apple : fruit
::
_______ : _______

desk : rectangle
::
_______ : _______

Texas : state
::
_______ : _______

pudding : soft
::
_______ : _______

United States : country
::
_______ : _______

glass : smooth
::
_______ : _______

green beans : vegetable
::
_______ : _______

shell : egg
::
__________ : __________

skyscraper : urban areas
::
__________ : __________

sandpaper : rough
::
__________ : __________

diamond : jewels
::
__________ : __________

grass : green
::
__________ : __________

puppy : pets
::
__________ : __________

sun : gas
::
__________ : __________

mail carrier : occupations
::
__________ : __________

scream : loud
::
__________ : __________

helicopter : transportation
::
__________ : __________

lemon : sour
::
__________ : __________

wide : narrow
::
__________ : __________

wing : bird
::
__________ : __________

fingernail : finger
::
__________ : __________

second : minute
::
__________ : __________

blood : person
::
__________ : __________

crust : pie
::
__________ : __________

trunk : tree
::
__________ : __________

tiger : stripes
::
__________ : __________

strings : guitar
::
__________ : __________

student : classroom
::
__________ : __________

computer : desk
::
__________ : __________

shark : ocean
::
__________ : __________

secretary : office
::
__________ : __________

Texan : Texas

::

__________ : __________

saddle : horse

::

__________ : __________

judge : courtroom

::

__________ : __________

watch : wrist

::

__________ : __________

door : lock

::

__________ : __________

tongue : taste

::

__________ : __________

fan : cool

::

__________ : __________

knife : cut

::

__________ : __________

artist : paint
::
__________ : __________

horn : honk
::
__________ : __________

ruler : measure
::
__________ : __________

book : read
::
__________ : __________

giggle : laugh
::
__________ : __________

yell : scream
::
__________ : __________

old : ancient
::
__________ : __________

strategy : plan
::
__________ : __________

aid : help

::

__________ : __________

ask : request

::

__________ : __________

ill : sick

::

__________ : __________

choice : option

::

__________ : __________

clean : dirty

::

__________ : __________

all : none

::

__________ : __________

above : below

::

__________ : __________

empty : full

::

__________ : __________

graceful : clumsy
::
_______ : _______

exciting : dull
::
_______ : _______

healthy : ill
::
_______ : _______

waiter : waitress
::
_______ : _______

calculator : add
::
_______ : _______

cold : freezing
::
_______ : _______

airplane : hanger
::
_______ : _______

_______ : _______
::
_______ : _______

WEIGH THE MEANING and DISCOVER THE PATTERN FOLLOW-UP ACTIVITIES

GOAL

To reinforce and review *Weigh the Meaning* and *Discover the Pattern* strategies

BACKGROUND INFORMATION

The main focus of this lesson is to review the previous two strategies. The strategy guide review pages will be compiled with similar pages into a booklet. This booklet, along with a vacation calendar, provides a means of practicing with family members and reinforcing skills throughout a school break. Although some educators may choose to do the strategy guide pages and homework activities at the end of each lesson, others prefer delayed reinforcement to strengthen knowledge of strategies, concepts, and vocabulary covered within the lessons. Using a small representation of the strategy poster, the strategy guide pages include the specific vocabulary from the lessons. An application component is provided on the second pages of the strategy guides. Students may do reflective writing about how the strategy is or can be useful to them.

OBJECTIVES

1. Tell and write the major components of the *Weigh the Meaning* and *Discover the Pattern* strategies.
2. Reflect and write about how the strategies will help at home, at school, and in the community.
3. Share strategy information with family members and complete the application activities.

MATERIALS

1. *Weigh the Meaning* poster (Created earlier)
2. *Discover the Pattern* poster (Created earlier)
3. *Weigh the Meaning Strategy Guide* (See pages 174–175; duplicate one per student.)
4. *Discover the Pattern Strategy Guide* (See pages 176–177; duplicate one per student.)
5. *Weigh the Meaning Homework Activity* (See page 178; duplicate one per student.)
6. *Discover the Pattern Homework Activity* (See page 179; duplicate one per student.)

INTRODUCTION

Tie-in to Prior Learning

Remind the students that they have now learned two more strategies that will help them move toward achieving their goals to improve their word power. Display and discuss the posters and strategies for these lessons. Have students tell about each of the strategies in their own words.

Focus/Relevancy

Review the importance of the *Strategy Guide Booklet* which will be a collection of the student's strategy guide pages for each strategy learned. The booklet will help them become better communicators by helping them remember all the strategies they will be learning. Remind students that new pages are added as new strategies are learned.

LESSON ACTIVITIES

1. Distribute the *Weigh the Meaning Strategy Guide* pages. Students are to demonstrate they know the strategy by completing the blank lines. Below the synonym scale, students are to write pairs of synonyms they know. Remind them to weigh the meaning of the words by putting the words in a sentence. If the meaning has stayed the same while making the sentence more interesting, the words are synonyms. Ask students to write the name of an excellent source for finding synonyms on their strategy guide page. (Write the word *thesaurus* on the board if necessary.)

2. On the lines beside the "Antonyms Are Opposites" heading, students are to write opposites they know. Encourage the students to practice the sentence strategy "It's not ____, it's ____" for antonyms. Have several students share their antonyms with the group. Compliment the students on the word power they have practiced so far.

3. On the second page of the strategy guide, have students write how this particular strategy has helped them or will help them at school, at home, or in the community. Brainstorm ideas (e.g., "I used synonyms to help me write a story for my reading class," "My friend and I played an antonym game and I did great").

4. Distribute the *Discover the Pattern Strategy Guide* pages. Review the strategy which stresses discovering the relationship pattern. Review the relationship patterns discussed (i.e., synonym, antonym, member/category, item/characteristic, part/whole, item/function, and item/location). Have a student study the first page of the strategy guide and summarize how to complete the activity. Make sure they point out that the choices are on the page. Notice that the last part of the analogy is blank. Students can also create their own analogies on a blank sheet of paper if they would like.

5. On the second page of the strategy guide, have students write how this particular strategy has helped them or will help them at school, at home, or in the community. Brainstorm ideas (e.g., "I know to look for patterns to help me solve problems I have").

6. Hand out the *Weigh the Meaning* and *Discover the Pattern Homework Activity* pages and discuss them. Reinforce the importance of sharing this information with family members, and the ease and fun of doing these assignments. They will only take a few minutes to complete, but students can impress their family with what they have learned! Have a reward system established to encourage students to bring their homework activity pages back to school signed by a family member.

CLOSURE

Summarize the lesson, review its relevance to students, and tie it to future learning. Discuss the objectives that were completed in this review (i.e., the students can tell and write the *Weigh the Same* and *Discover the Pattern* strategies; they can tell how they will use the strategies; they know the strategies well enough to share them with their family members).

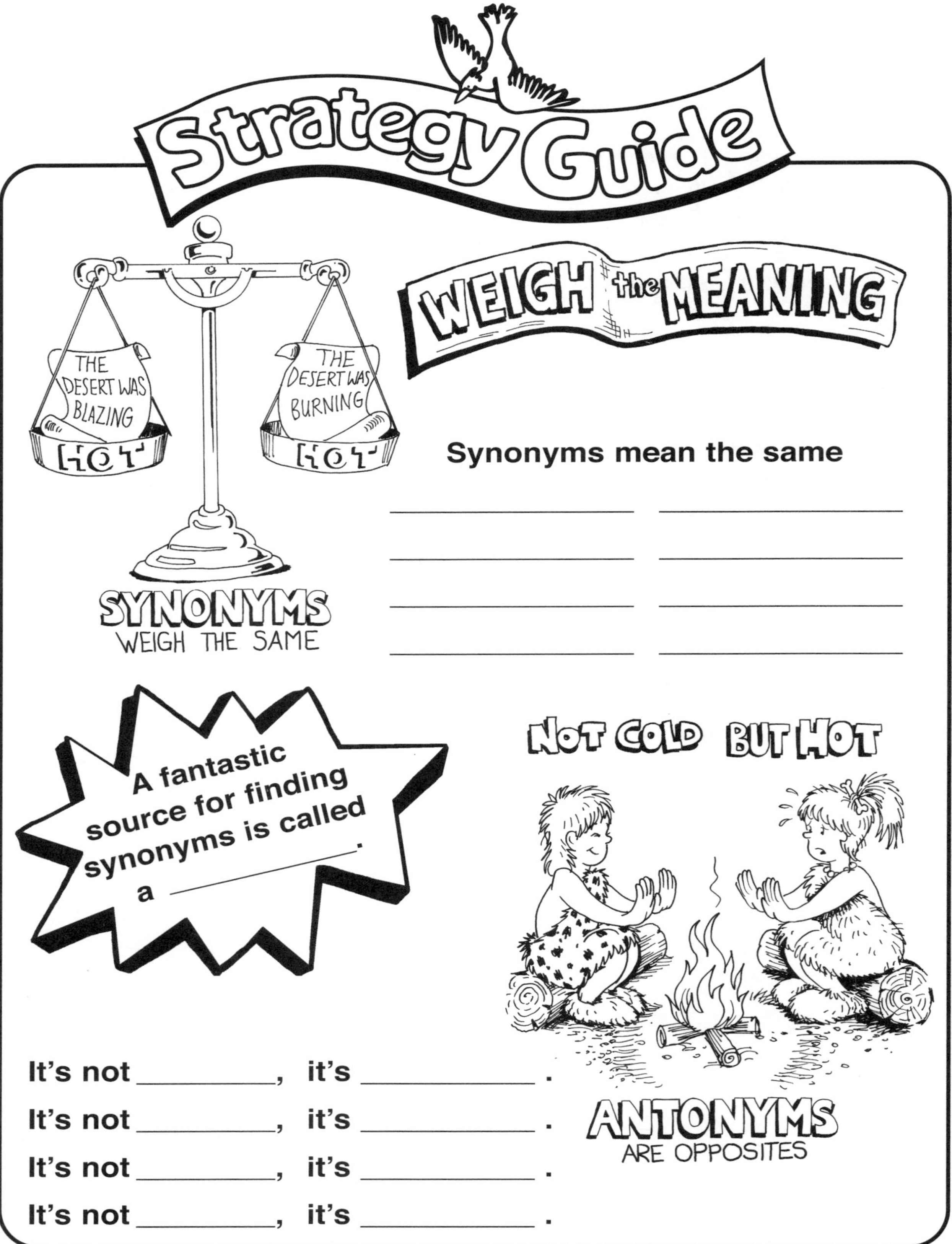
Strategy Guide
WEIGH the MEANING
THE DESERT WAS BLAZING
HOT
THE DESERT WAS BURNING
HOT
SYNONYMS
WEIGH THE SAME
Synonyms mean the same
A fantastic source for finding synonyms is called a ______________.
NOT COLD BUT HOT
ANTONYMS
ARE OPPOSITES
It's not __________, it's ____________ .
It's not __________, it's ____________ .
It's not __________, it's ____________ .
It's not __________, it's ____________ .

Weigh the Meaning: Synonyms and Antonyms

Name: ______________________________ Date: ______________

Directions: Write a sentence about how you have used or will use the strategy in each place.

At home, I ______________________________

____

____

____

____

____

At school, I ______________________________

____

____

____

____

____

In my community, I ______________________________

____

____

____

____

____

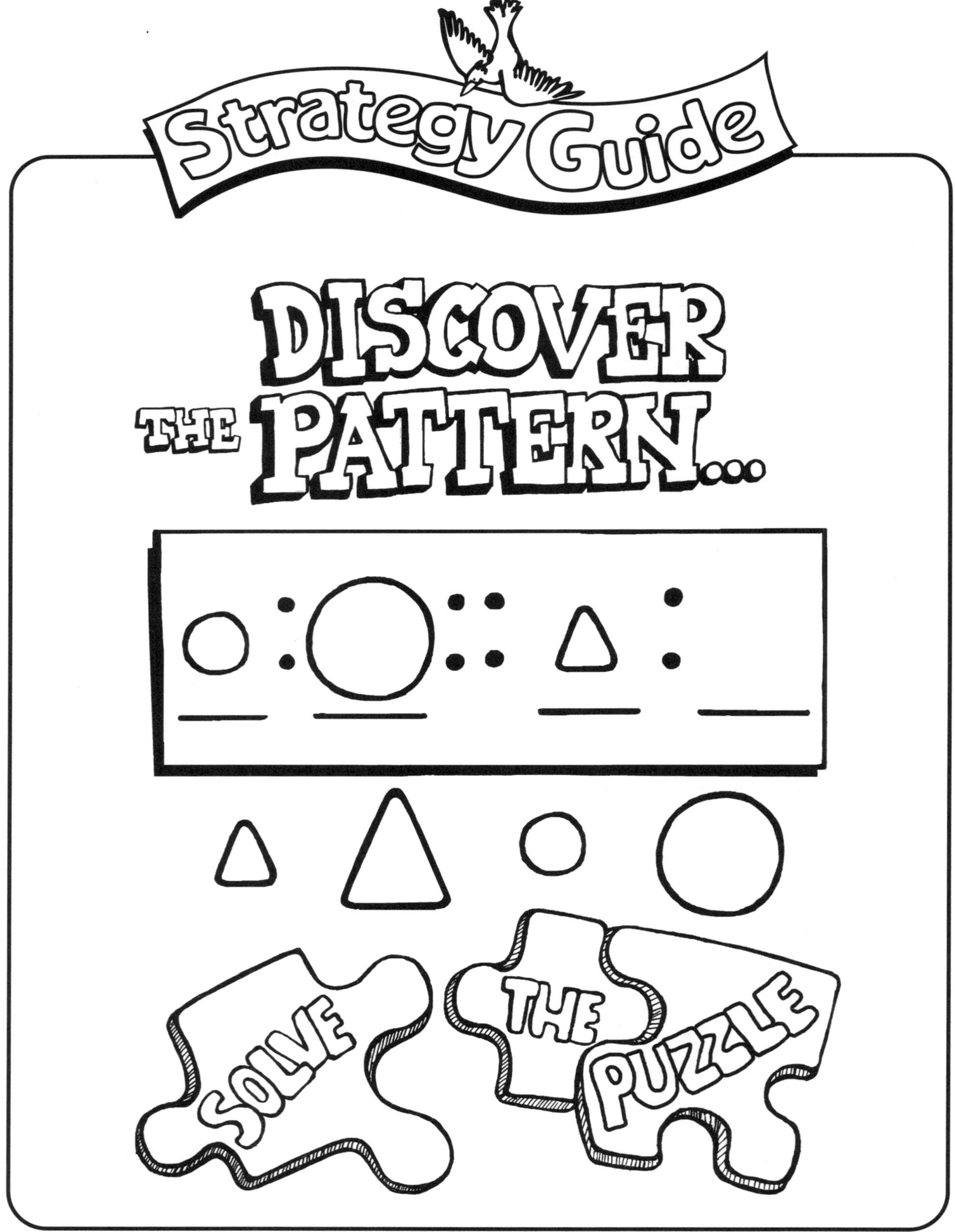
Strategy Guide
DISCOVER
THE PATTERN...
SOLVE
THE
PUZZLE

Discover the Pattern: Analogies

Name: ______________________ Date: __________

Directions: Write a sentence about how you have used or will use the strategy in each place.

At home, I ______________________

At school, I ______________________

In my community, I ______________________

Homework Activity

WEIGH the MEANING
NOT COLD BUT HOT
THE DESERT WAS BLAZING
THE DESERT WAS BURNING
HOT
HOT
SYNONYMS
WEIGH THE SAME
ANTONYMS
ARE OPPOSITES

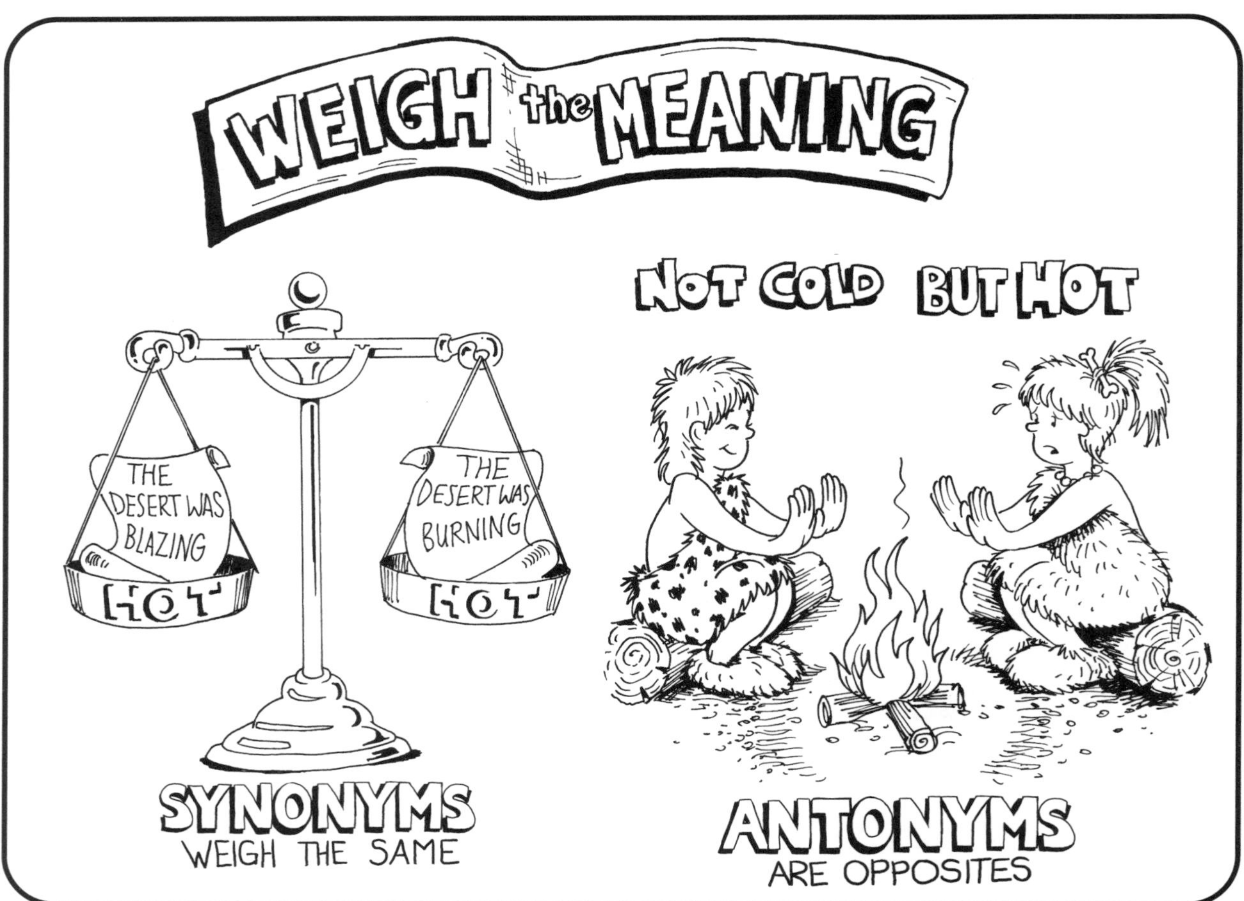

Dear Family,

1. Have your child explain the *Weigh the Meaning* strategy and tell why it's important to know how to use synonyms and antonyms.
2. Play a synonym game by telling your child a sentence and having him or her use a synonym for one of the words you used. Here are some examples:
   The stove felt *hot* when I touched it. The ice cube was *cold* in my hand.
   Mother said the TV was too *loud.* I was *happy* when I got my new shoes.
3. Play an antonym game by giving your child a word and having him or her tell you the opposite of the word. Here are some example words:
   right-left high-low sweet-sour
4. If your child completes these activities, please sign below and return this form to school.

Family Member: ______________________________ Date: ____________________

Homework Activity

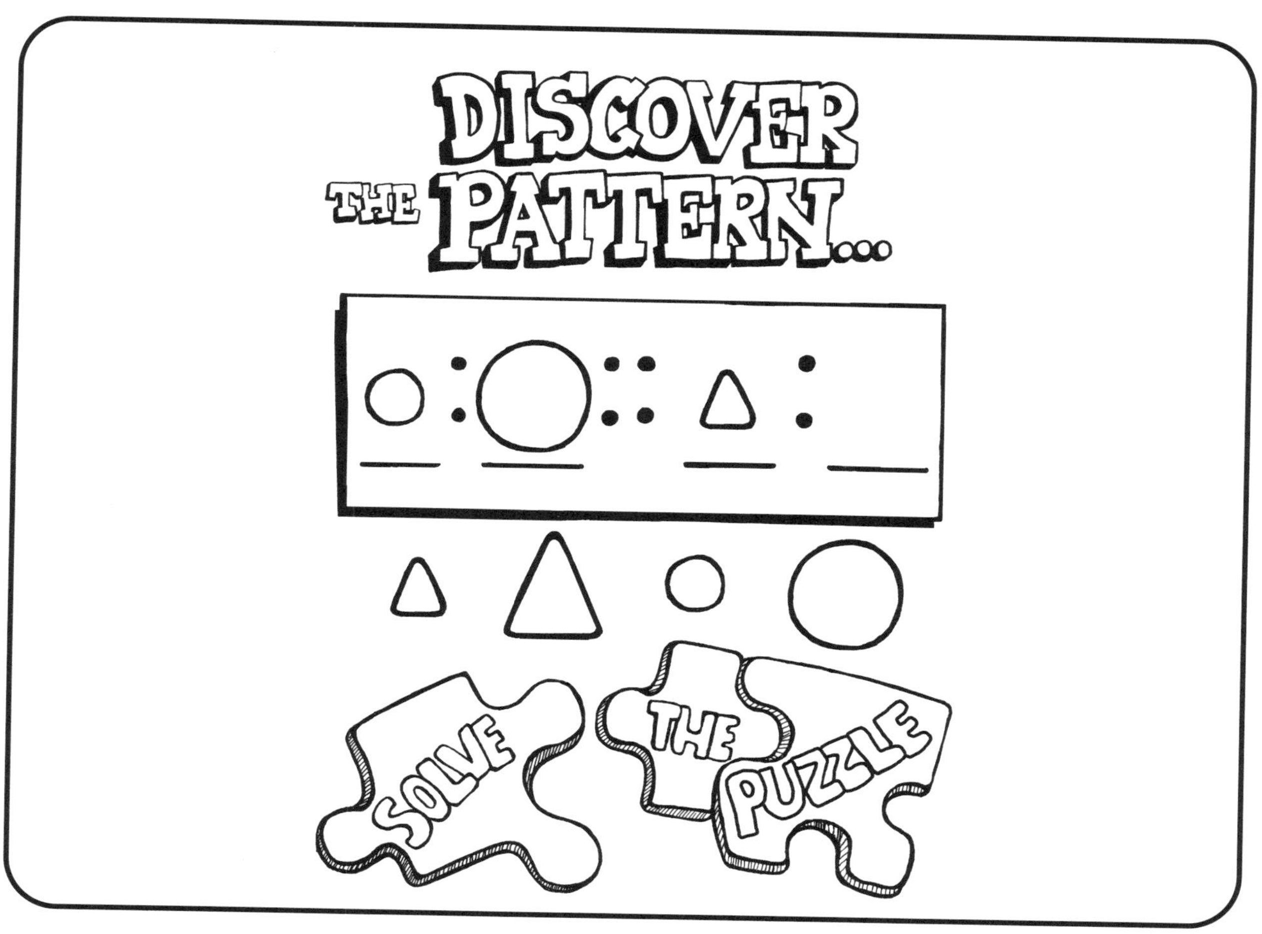

Dear Family,

1. Have your child explain the *Discover the Pattern* strategy and tell how looking for a pattern can help them solve analogies.
2. Have your child explain the symbols used in analogies.
3. Have your child create an analogy for you to solve. Here are some starter analogies:

   ceiling : floor :: inside : ______
   knife : sharp :: refrigerator : _____
   stick : nest :: brick : ______
   gift : present :: ill : _____

4. If your child completes these activities, please sign below and return this form to school.

Family Member: ______________________ Date: ______________

FOCUS FOR CLARITY: DEFINITIONS

GOAL

To define words clearly and precisely

BACKGROUND INFORMATION

The main emphasis of the *Focus for Clarity* strategy is to help students be aware of what makes a clear and precise definition and to use this information when defining words. This lesson relies on the students' knowledge of a number of other strategies, especially those developing their word power, categorization, and description skills (i.e., *It Makes Sense, Lasso the Word Herd, Weigh the Meaning,* and *Compare Contrastadon*). The previously learned strategies will help students organize their thoughts into a clear, precise definition. Students are taught that a clear definition includes a label or name, a category, and a distinctive feature of the word being defined. These elements of a definition apply primarily to definitions of nouns.

Parts of speech are referred to in this lesson. These include nouns, verbs, and adjectives. These concepts may need to be reviewed, pretaught, or adapted, depending on the level of students. Therefore, this lesson may require more than one session. Also, the students create a cinquain (pronounced sĭng´ kān) poem as a strategy for remembering the elements of a good definition. The creation of the cinquain poem may also require more than one session. Students really enjoy the opportunity to create and share their poems and illustrations and should be given sufficient time to do this.

OBJECTIVES

1. Identify information that makes a definition clear and precise.
2. Identify parts of speech as they pertain to defining words.
3. Write a definition using a cinquain poem format.
4. Define a word using the elements of a clear definition.

MATERIALS

1. *Focus for Clarity* graphic (See page 185; duplicate and enlarge the graphic, color it, mount it onto poster board, and laminate it for durability, if desired.)
2. Chalkboard and chalk
3. *The Great Kapok Tree* (1990) by Lynne Cherry (If desired, substitute another book. This book was selected because of the beautiful illustrations of both familiar and unusual animals that reside in a rainforest environment. The story lends itself to discussions about ecology, geography, and people's responsibility to the world environment. A number of different language concepts can be emphasized.)

4. *Brainstorm* (See page 186; duplicate one per small group.)
5. *Cinquain Pattern* (See page 187; duplicate one per student.)

INTRODUCTION

Tie-in to Prior Learning

Refer to the growth in word power that the students have demonstrated and explain that they will be continuing to develop and use their word power as they learn about telling and writing definitions.

Focus/Relevancy

1. Show the *Focus for Clarity* poster. Ask students what they think a definition is and discuss their responses. Refer to the poster and ask how many students have ever taken a picture. Ask what happens if the camera moves as the picture is snapped (i.e., the resulting picture will be unclear and blurry). Pantomime the action of focusing the lens of a camera while asking what a photographer is doing when he turns the lens of the camera. Say to students,

   You turn the lens to focus on an object. You want your picture to be sharp and clear. Defining a word is like focusing a camera. We want the definition to be sharp and clear so the listener or reader understands what you mean.

2. To illustrate the need for clear and precise definitions, intentionally model an imprecise and unclear definition while drawing parts of an animal on the board. As you draw, say to the students,

   I'm going to give you the definition of what I'm drawing while I draw a picture on the board. See if you get a clear picture of what I'm defining.

   - *It's an animal.* (Draw an oval shape on the board.) *Do you know what animal I'm defining?* (Encourage students to generate some possibilities.) *Apparently I am not being clear enough! You must need more information!*
   - *It has four legs.* (Add four large legs to your drawing. Let students generate some more possibilities. Discuss how it is often helpful when problem solving to eliminate possible alternatives.) *This creature has a large body and four big legs so we know it cannot be a snake. Name another animal that it cannot be. Do you need more information?*
   - *It's a jungle animal.* (Add a circular head to the drawing and discuss what it could and could not be.) *I need to tell you something unique or distinctive about this animal to make my definition clearer.*

- *This animal has large ears and a trunk and it likes to eat peanuts.* (Add ears and a trunk to your drawing. At this point, students should recognize the drawing as an elephant. Point out that once you added the distinctive feature of the animal, everyone clearly knew what was being defined.) *A good definition makes the meaning as clear as a photograph.*

3. Discuss that in this lesson, students will be using a number of the important communication strategies they have already learned and applying them to telling and writing definitions. The strategy learned in this lesson will help them define words that are places or things (i.e., nouns) but they can apply the idea of being clear and precise when they define any type of word. Have students give examples of when they have had to define words at school (e.g., spelling, reading, social studies, science, physical education, etc.). Most of the time, students will need to know and tell the meaning in their own words.

LESSON ACTIVITIES

1. Discuss the problem with the imprecise definition given as an example during *Focus/Relevancy* (e.g., pieces of information were shared a little at a time, but not the most important information). Stress that a clear, precise definition (of a place or thing) must include these elements:
   - the label or name (elephant)
   - the category (jungle animal)
   - a distinctive feature(s)
2. Remind students that they learned about distinctive features in the *Creature Creator* lesson and in a definition, the distinctive feature might be what the thing being defined looks like (appearance) or what the thing being defined does. In the case of the elephant example, the distinctive features were the large ears, trunk, and the fact that it eats peanuts.
3. Model giving a complete definition of the elephant using all of the elements: An elephant is a jungle animal that has large ears, a trunk, and eats peanuts.
4. Explain that the students will be writing definitions of animals mentioned in the story *The Great Kapok Tree.* Encourage the students to use their listening skills to help them choose the animal they want to write about as they hear the story.
5. Before reading the story, highlight the literary components (see page 12). Discuss the author, illustrator and unique vocabulary.

6. Begin to read the story. While reading, point out the following literary highlights:
   - Vocabulary—Define *lulled, gash, generations, ancestors, pollen/pollinate, canopy, wither, underbrush, smoldering, dappled, rare, dangle, suspended, fragrant.*
   - Figurative language—Discuss *tree of miracles, feast your eyes, look upon us with new eyes.*
7. Finish reading the story. After reading the story, remind students that they will need to choose an animal from the story to use in their definition.
8. Write the following cinquain poem on the board; talk about each line and the type of words that are used:

   Kapok
   Giant, Strong
   Growing, Swaying, Sheltering
   Home to many creatures
   Tree

   Using this example, discuss the parts of speech that are used in each line of the poem. Ask the students if they are familiar with the following parts of speech.

   noun (label)—the name of the place or thing
   adjective—describing word
   verb—action word with *-ing* ending
   four-word phrase telling a unique or distinctive feature
   synonym—another word that means the same thing; or category name (if no synonym)

   Review or explain as needed.
9. Explain to students how the form of a cinquain is part of its definition. Write the following on the board next to the Kapok tree cinquain:

   Noun
   Adjective, Adjective
   Verb(ing), Verb(ing), Verb(ing)
   Four-word phrase telling distinctive feature
   Synonym (or category name)
10. Break students into small groups of three or four. Hand out the *Brainstorm* activity sheet and discuss how brainstorming means listing as many ideas as possible for later use. Instruct the

groups to choose their favorite animal from the story and write the name of the animal on the "Label or Name" line. Groups should complete the sheet by brainstorming words that describe their animal and writing them in the appropriate brain (e.g., the "doing verbs" are written in the "verbs" brain). Explain that they will be using some of their ideas to create a cinquain poem about their animal.

11. Hand out the *Cinquain Pattern* activity sheet to each student. Direct the small groups to choose their best or favorite words from their *Brainstorm* activity sheet to complete the *Cinquain Pattern*. Rather than using a synonym for the last line, the students should use the category name to keep the essential parts of a definition. Students can agree on the cinquain as a group or each create their own but each student should complete a cinquain. Encourage each student to add an illustration of the animal to their cinquain.

    HINT

    This activity may also be completed by student pairs.

12. Have students share their cinquains with the large group. As a last step, have each student give a clear and precise definition of their animal.

13. To add more challenge to this activity, have students use the elements of a definition to define a new word they have learned in another class.

CLOSURE

Summarize the lesson, review its relevance to students, and tie it to future learning. Congratulate the students on their animal definitions, which were written in a different way by putting them into a poem. Stress that the important thing to remember when telling or writing a definition (of a noun) for any subject is to include the label, the category, and the unique or distinctive features. Have each student think of one situation when they have had to define a noun.

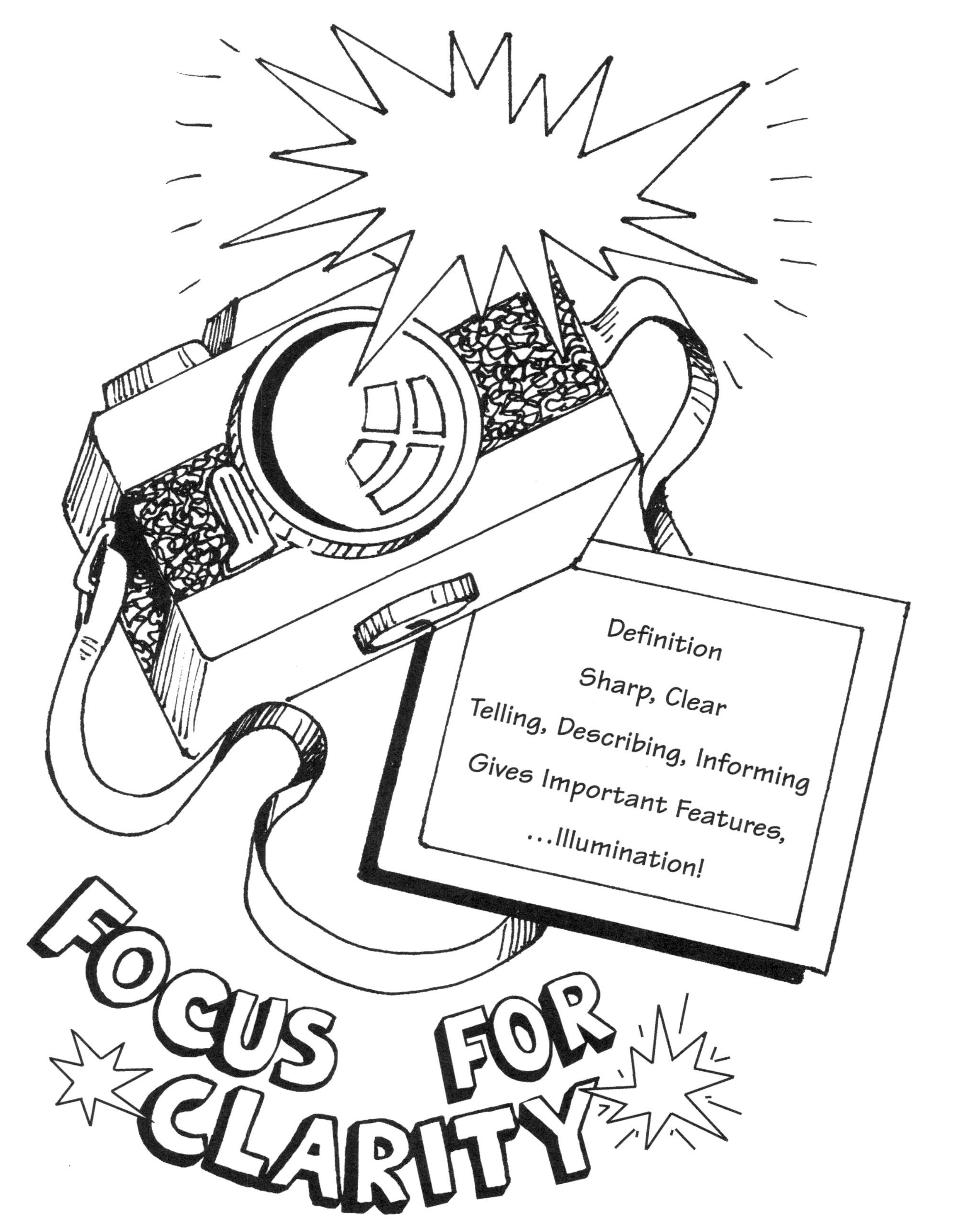
Definition
Sharp, Clear
Telling, Describing, Informing
Gives Important Features,
...Illumination!
FOCUS FOR CLARITY

Brainstorm

Names: ____

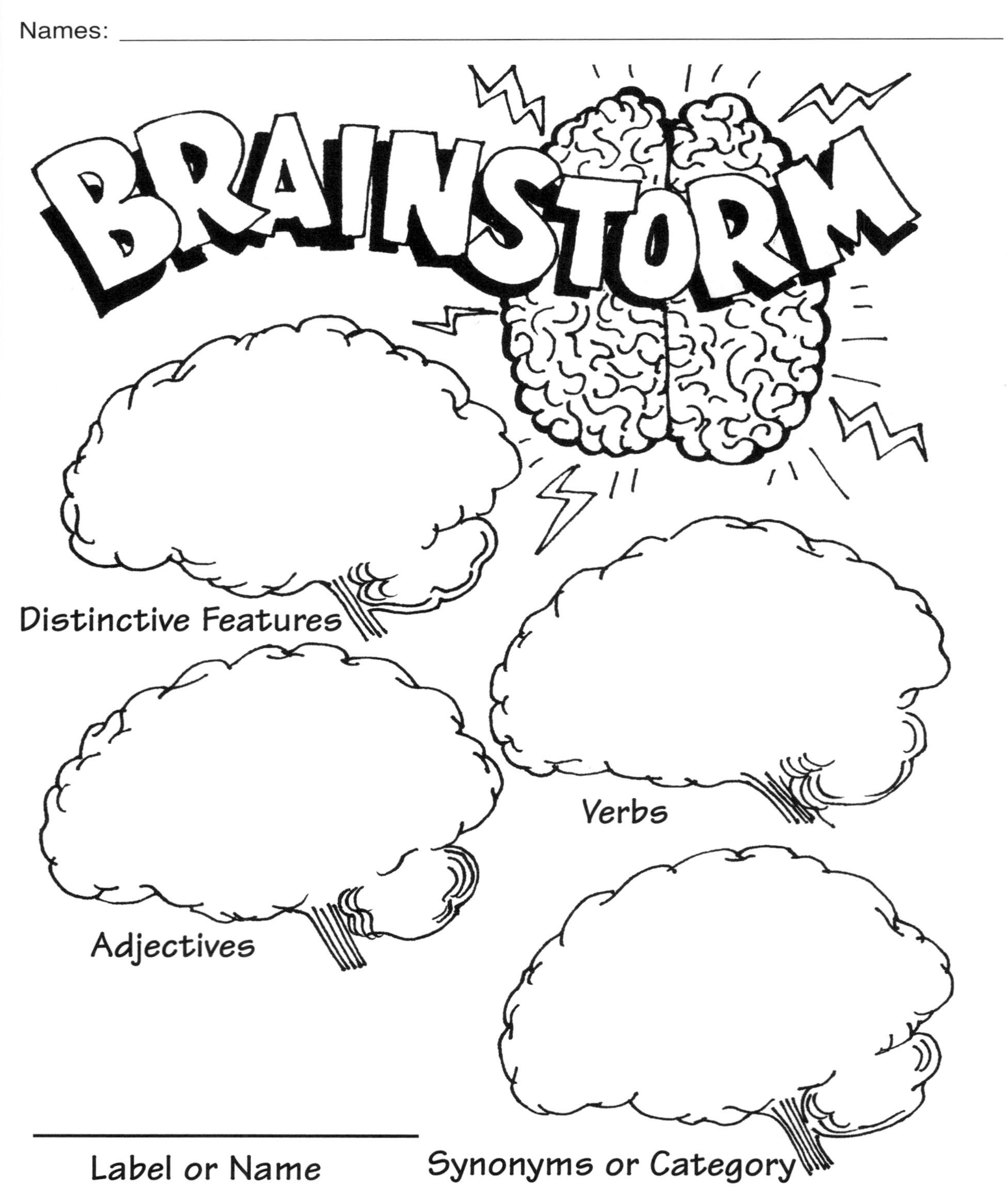

Cinquain Pattern

Names: ____________________

____

____
noun (label)

____________ ____________
(adjective) (adjective)

____________ ____________ ____________
verb(ing) verb(ing) verb(ing)

____________ ____________ ____________ ____________
four words telling feature

____
synonym (or category)

CHAMELEON WORDS: WORDS WITH MULTIPLE MEANING

GOAL

To identify and use words with multiple meaning

BACKGROUND INFORMATION

The main focus of the *Chameleon Words* strategy is to help students recognize and use context clues to determine the intended meaning of a word with multiple meanings. *Multiple meaning words* are words that have more than one meaning or referent. The ability to understand and use multiple meaning words is basic to understanding figurative language (Gorman-Gard, 1992). And Wiig and Semel (1980) found usage of multiple meaning words in academic classroom materials to be staggering.

In this lesson, double function words (i.e., words that have a physical and psychological referent) are considered multiple meaning words. But the educator should be aware that children do not connect the physical and psychological relationship until age 9 or 10 (Asch and Nerlove, 1960) and should avoid these words (e.g., sweet, hard) if using this lesson with younger students. This lesson also considers homophones to be chameleon words.

This lesson includes identifying parts of speech, categorization, and labeling, as prerequisite skills.

OBJECTIVES

1. Identify and name words that have more than one meaning.
2. Recognize and use context clues to explain the intended meaning of a word with multiple meaning.

MATERIALS

1. Chalkboard and chalk
2. *Chameleon Words* graphic (See page 192; duplicate and enlarge the graphic, color it, mount it onto poster board, and laminate it for durability, if desired.)
3. *Eye Spy* (1991) by Linda Bourke (If desired, substitute another book. This book was selected because it provides an entertaining look at the multiple meanings of words. The students enjoy trying to guess the next word from the clues in the last picture on each page.)
4. *Multiple Meaning Madness* (See page 193; duplicate one per small group.)

INTRODUCTION

Tie-in to Prior Learning

Review the elements needed in a clear and precise definition: label or name, category, and distinctive features. Remind students these elements help a listener or reader picture the word being defined. Tell them that some words have more than one definition or meaning and that is what this strategy is about.

Focus/Relevancy

1. Ask for a volunteer to come to the board to spell a word. Ask the student to write the word *meet*. If the student asks for more information before writing, compliment him or her on recognizing the need, and prompt the student to ask about the context (e.g.,"Do you mean the meat that we eat, a swim meet, or to meet someone after school?"). If the student does not ask for clarification and simply writes one form of the word on the board, ask the student if he or she is sure of the spelling. Elicit the need to request clarification. Highlight the need to hear the word in context to know exactly which word to write. Explain that context means putting the word into a sentence that will give enough information to know the correct spelling or meaning.

2. Stress that many words have more that one meaning and learning how to recognize these different intended meanings will help them avoid confusion.

LESSON ACTIVITIES

1. Show the *Chameleon Words* poster to prepare for teaching the concept of context. Say to students,

   Who can tell me something about a chameleon? Chameleons have the ability to change their color according to their surroundings. We are going to talk about chameleon words. Some chameleon words are pen, by, new, fair. *Why do you think we call them* chameleon words? (Give students a chance to respond.) *These words change their meaning depending on their surroundings or the context.*

2. Compare the meanings of the word *wave* by referring to the symbols on the poster which mean "The wave crashed on the shore," "I wave to my friends when I say hello." Relate the change in meaning in each context to the change of a chameleon to its surroundings. Highlight the multiple meaning word in each sentence and point out the other words that make-up the surroundings or context.

3. Refer to the poster to illustrate that identifying how the word is used can also help determine word meaning. Discuss how the word *wave* can be used as a noun (person, place, or thing) or as a verb (action).

4. Show the book *Eye Spy*. Before reading the story, tell students that they will need to figure out the chameleon words pictured in the book and to explain their meanings by using the word in

a sentence context (e.g., for the word *fly* there is a picture of a fishing fly and a pop fly in a baseball game. The student would need to use *fly* in an appropriate sentence such as "The batter hit a pop fly in the eighth inning").

HINT

An optional activity would be to tell all the parts of speech the multiple meaning word could represent. Then have students tally the number of noun, verb, and adjective meanings for each of the pictures in the book. This allows students to give additional meanings for the words if all meanings are not pictured in the book (e.g., for the word *fly*, the insect meaning is not pictured).

5. After telling the students what to look for in the book, highlight the literary components (see page 12). Discuss the author and the illustrator.

6. Begin to read the book by looking at the pictures. Continually remind the students that the word may be used as a noun or verb and occasionally as an adjective. They need to ask themselves, "Is it a person, place, or thing? Is it something I can do? Does it describe something?" The students enjoy trying to guess the next word from the clues in the last picture on each page.

7. Divide into small groups. Distribute one *Multiple Meaning Madness* activity page to each group. Have each group brainstorm as many meanings as they can for each word on their *Multiple Meaning Madness* activity page. They must write a phrase that supplies a context to show the meaning (e.g., key in the door, key of the map, key to the mystery, piano key). Remind students that they can change the spelling of the word as the meaning changes for words that are homophones. Have each group tally the number of meanings for each word. Have the group with the most meanings share their sentences. Have other groups add to this if they have additional meanings. Challenge each group to complete the activity sheet by thinking of another word that has multiple meanings.

8. This lesson can be extended through the use of jokes and humor. The humor of many riddles and cartoons is based on words with multiple meanings. Refer students to the *Amelia Bedelia* books by Peggy Parish or other joke or riddle books available from a library. As an extension of this lesson, allow several students for the next several class meetings to share a riddle with the class. Do this until all students have had a turn to tell a riddle.

CLOSURE

Summarize the lesson, review its relevance to students, and tie it to future learning. Stress that multiple meaning words can help expand vocabulary and build word power. Knowing chameleon words can also be fun because they can be used to tell jokes and entertain others. A place where multiple meaning words are used frequently is in the sports world. Have each student find one multiple meaning word in the sports section of a newspaper and tell at least two meanings for the word.

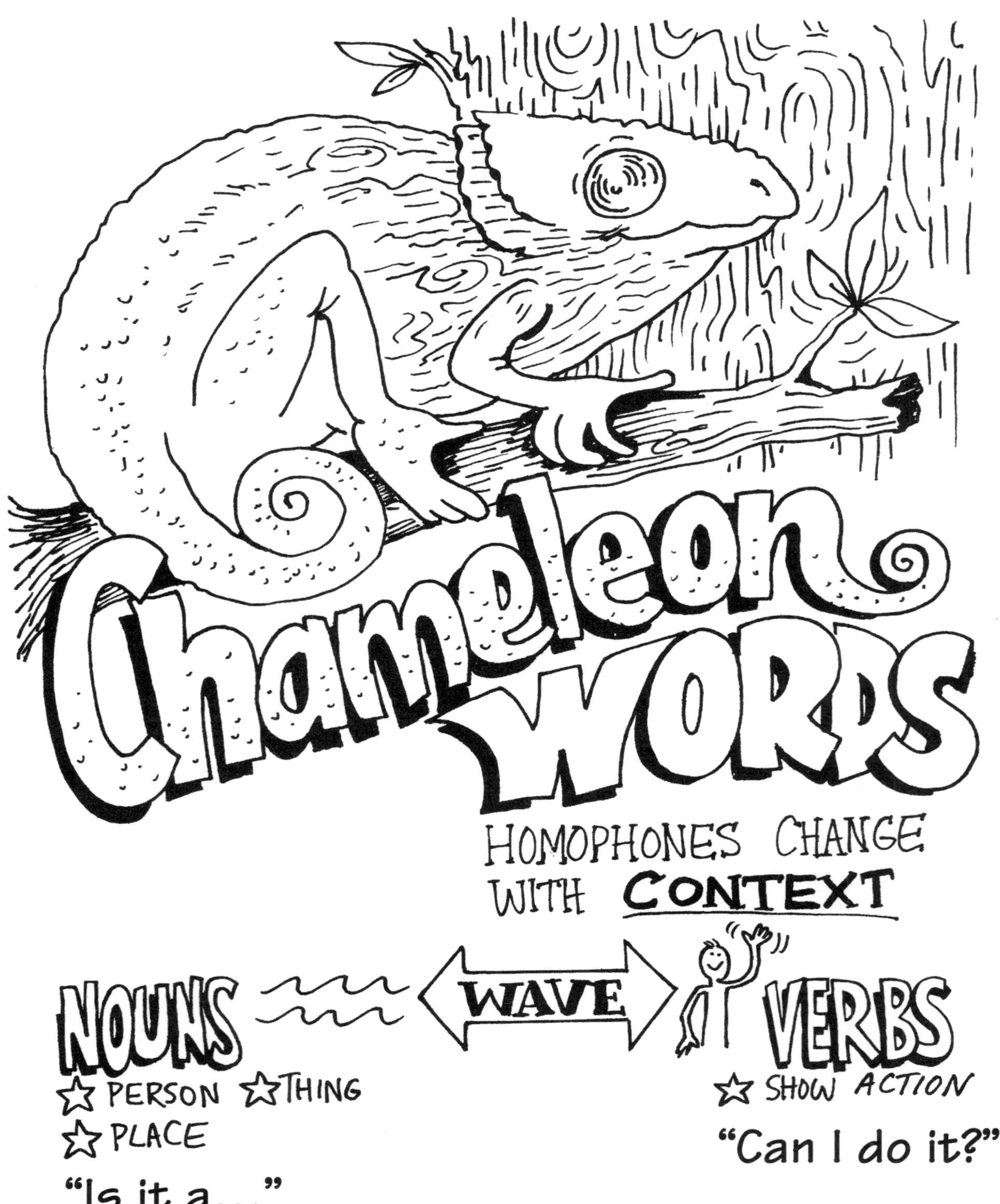
Chameleon WORDS
HOMOPHONES CHANGE WITH CONTEXT
NOUNS
WAVE
VERBS
☆ PERSON ☆ THING
☆ PLACE
"Is it a..."
☆ SHOW ACTION
"Can I do it?"

MULTIPLE MEANING madness

Names: ____

____

Directions: Think of as many meanings as you can for each word. Write a sentence or phrase to use the word in context. Then count the number of meanings you have for each word and write it on the "Total" line. Choose your own multiple meaning word for the last frame.

key

Total __________

pen

Total __________

map

Total __________

write

Total __________

pop

Total __________

____
write your own

Total __________

FOCUS FOR CLARITY and CHAMELEON WORDS FOLLOW-UP ACTIVITIES

GOAL

To reinforce and review *Focus for Clarity* and *Chameleon Words* strategies

BACKGROUND INFORMATION

The main focus of this lesson is to review the previous two strategies. The strategy guide review pages will be compiled with similar pages into a booklet. This booklet, along with a vacation calendar, provide a means of practicing with family members and reinforcing skills throughout a school break. Although some educators may choose to do the strategy guide pages and homework activities at the end of each lesson, others prefer delayed reinforcement to strengthen knowledge of strategies, concepts, and vocabulary covered within the lessons. Using a small representation of the strategy poster, the strategy guide pages include the specific vocabulary from the lessons. An application component is provided on the second pages of the strategy guides. Students may do reflective writing about how the strategy is or can be useful to them.

OBJECTIVES

1. Tell and write the major components of the *Focus for Clarity* and *Chameleon Words* strategies.
2. Reflect and write about how the strategies will help at home, at school, and in the community.
3. Share strategy information with family members and complete the application activities.

MATERIALS

1. *Focus for Clarity* poster (Created earlier)
2. *Chameleon Words* poster (Created earlier)
3. *Focus for Clarity Strategy Guide* (See pages 197–198; duplicate one per student.)
4. *Chameleon Words Strategy Guide* (See pages 199–200; duplicate one per student.)
5. *Focus for Clarity Homework Activity* (See page 201; duplicate one per student.)
6. *Chameleon Words Homework Activity* (See page 202; duplicate one per student.)

INTRODUCTION

Tie-in to Prior Learning

Remind the students that they have now learned two more strategies that will help them move toward achieving their goals to improve their word power. Display and discuss the posters and strategies for these lessons. Have students tell about each of the strategies in their own words.

Focus/Relevancy

Review the importance of the *Strategy Guide Booklet* which will be a collection of the student's strategy guide pages for each strategy learned. The booklet will help them become better communicators by helping them remember all the strategies they will be learning. Remind students that new pages are added as new strategies are learned.

LESSON ACTIVITIES

1. Distribute the *Focus for Clarity Strategy Guide* pages. Students are to demonstrate they know the strategy by completing the activity on the first page of the strategy guide. Give each student a noun to define. Using a word from the curriculum will help to generalize strategy use. Refer to the poster and have it displayed for the students.

2. On the second page of the *Focus for Clarity Strategy Guide,* have students write how this particular strategy has helped them or will help them at school, at home, or in the community. Brainstorm ideas (e.g., "I have to define words in my spelling assignment today," "My Mom asked me what an *ewok* was and I knew how to define it for her," "I was in the toy store and a clerk asked me what I was looking for and I had to define the toy because I forgot the name of it").

3. Distribute the *Chameleon Words Strategy Guide* pages and have students complete them. Students should demonstrate they know the strategy by completing the activity on the first page of the strategy guide. Refer to the poster and have it displayed for the students. Remind the students about words from the *Eye Spy* book and talk about the use of context to show meaning. Review the use of parts of speech when giving multiple meanings of words. Have students write phrases to show the different meanings of the words listed. Have students share their phrases.

4. On the second page of the *Chameleon Words Strategy Guide,* have students write how this particular strategy has helped them or will help them at school, at home, or in the community. Brainstorm ideas (e.g., "My Mom told me a riddle and it made me laugh because I knew the word had two meanings," "At the baseball game, the announcer said that the hit was good and I knew what he meant by *hit,*" "In the book I'm reading, I knew what the author meant when he used the word *lightweight*").

5. Hand out the *Focus for Clarity* and the *Chameleon Words Homework Activity* pages and discuss them. Reinforce the importance of sharing this information with family members, and the ease and fun of doing these assignments. They will only take a few minutes to complete, but students can impress their family with what they have learned! Have a reward system established to

encourage students to bring their homework activity pages back to school signed by a family member.

CLOSURE

Summarize the lesson, review its relevance to students, and tie it to future learning. Discuss the objectives that were completed in this review (i.e., the students can tell and write the *Focus for Clarity* and the *Chameleon Words* strategies; they can tell how they will use the strategies; they know the strategies well enough to share them with their family members).

Strategy Guide
Definition
Sharp, Clear
Telling, Describing, Informing
Gives Important Features,
...Illumination!
FOCUS FOR CLARITY

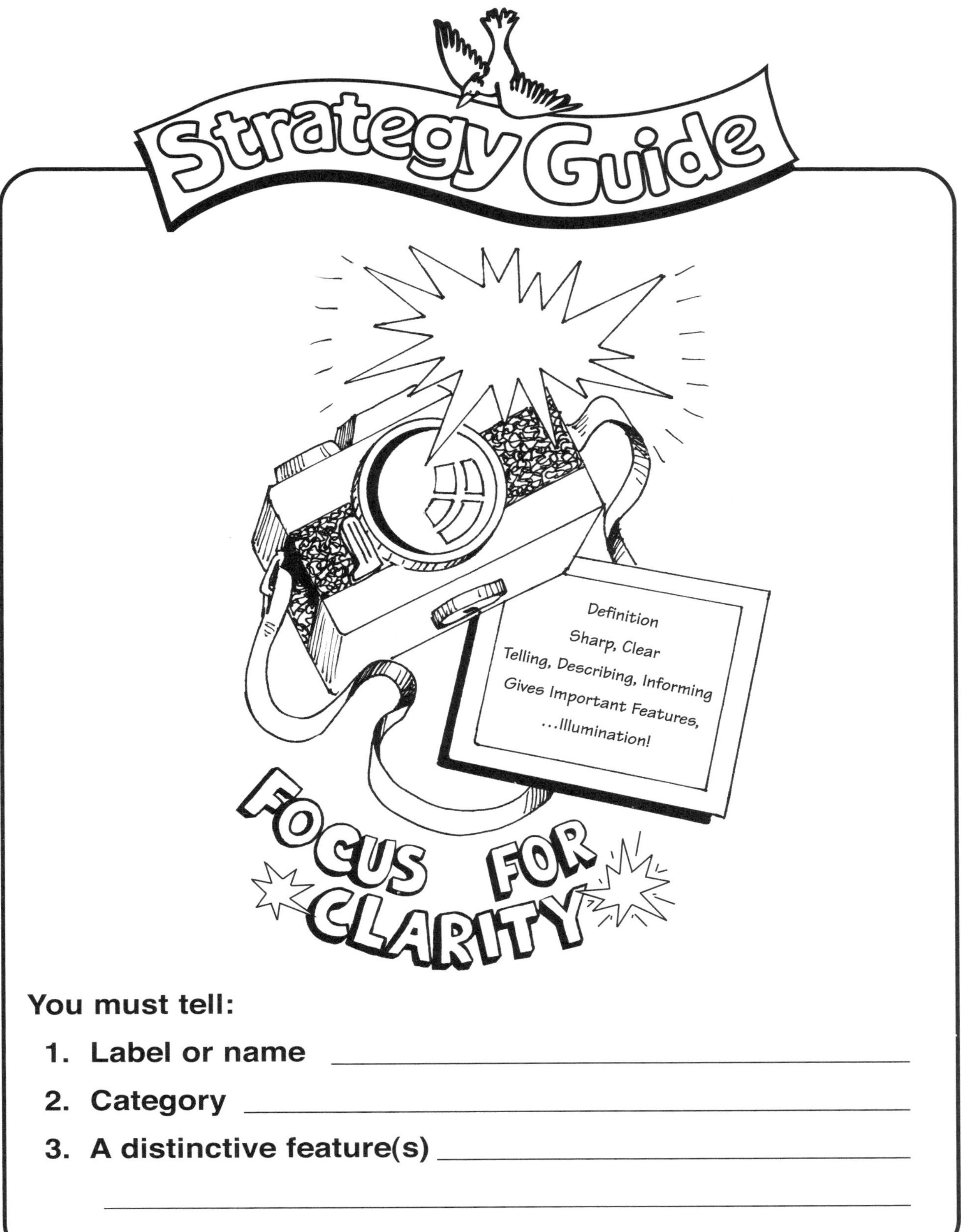

You must tell:

1. **Label or name** ______________________________
2. **Category** ______________________________
3. **A distinctive feature(s)** ______________________________

____

Focus for Clarity: Definitions

Name: ________________________ Date: ____________

Directions: Write a sentence about how you have used or will use the strategy in each place.

At home, I ______________________________

____

____

____

____

____

At school, I ______________________________

____

____

____

____

____

In my community, I ______________________________

____

____

____

____

____

Strategy Guide
Chameleon WORDS
HOMOPHONES CHANGE WITH CONTEXT
NOUNS
WAVE
VERBS
☆ PERSON ☆ THING
☆ PLACE
"Is it a..."
☆ SHOW ACTION
"Can I do it?"

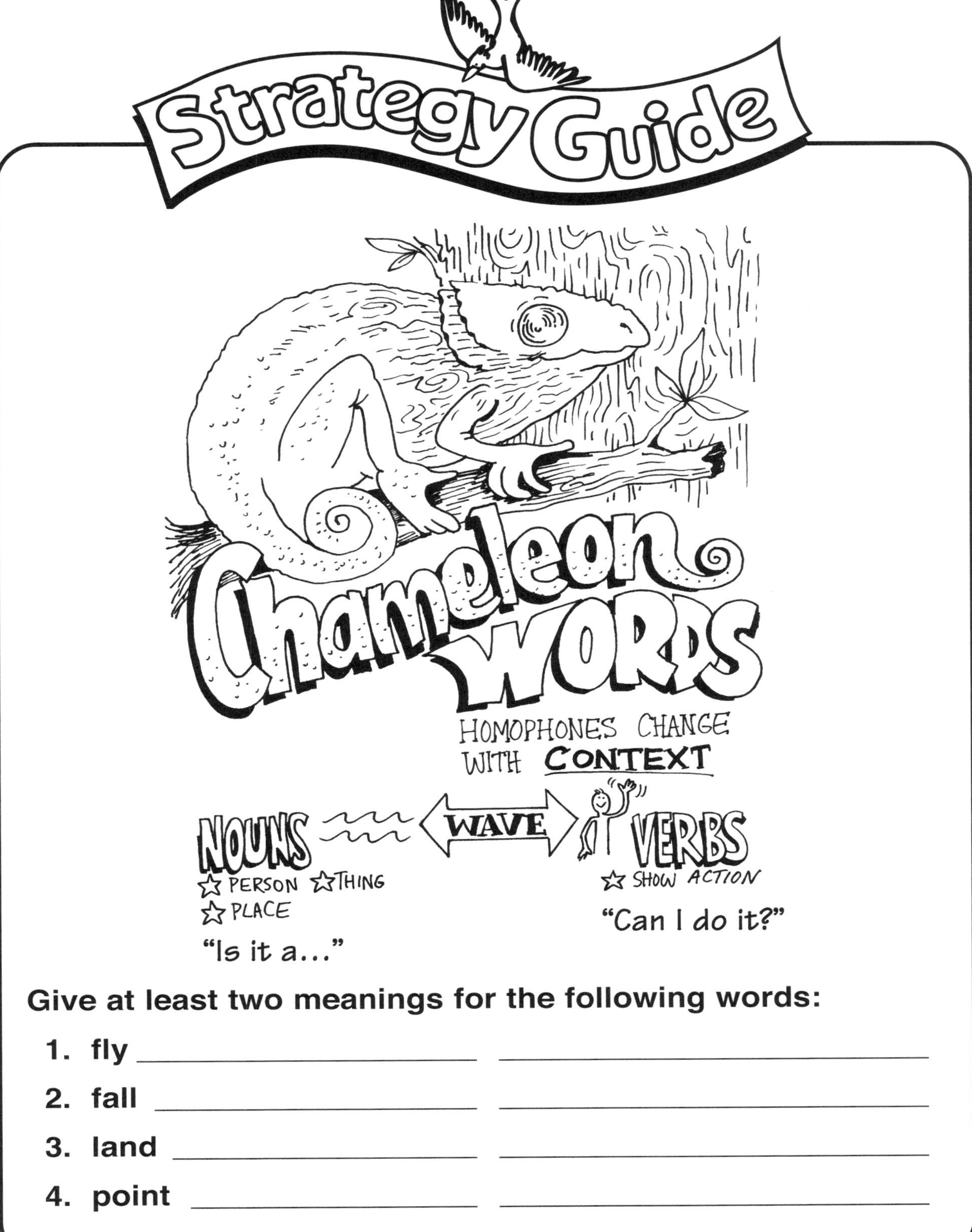

Give at least two meanings for the following words:

1. **fly** ____________________ ____________________
2. **fall** ____________________ ____________________
3. **land** ____________________ ____________________
4. **point** ____________________ ____________________

Chameleon Words: Words with Multiple Meaning

Name: ______________________________ Date: ______________

Directions: Write a sentence about how you have used or will use the strategy in each place.

At home, I ______________________________

____

____

____

____

____

At school, I ______________________________

____

____

____

____

____

In my community, I ______________________________

____

____

____

____

____

Homework Activity

Definition
Sharp, Clear
Telling, Describing, Informing
Gives Important Features,
...Illumination!
FOCUS FOR CLARITY

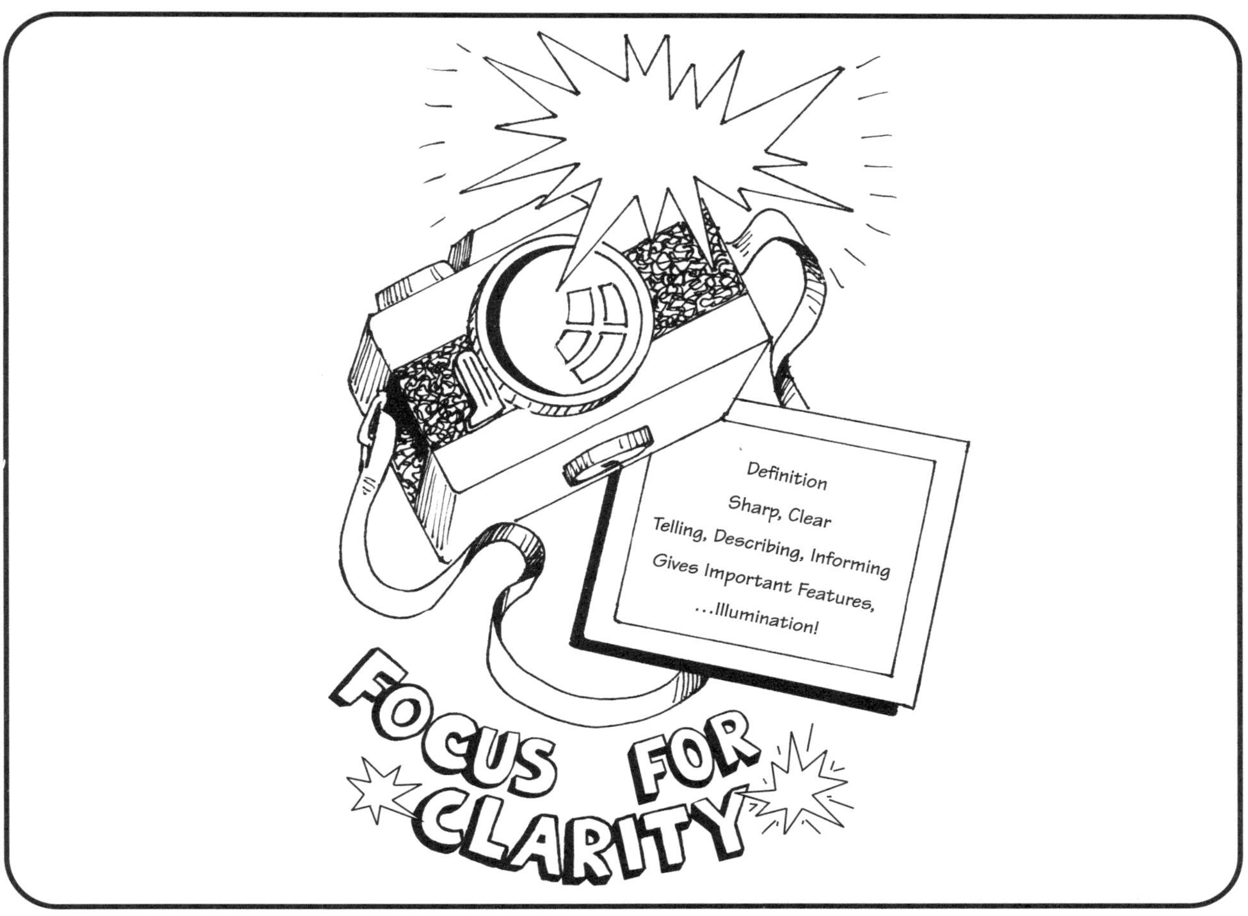

Dear Family,

1. Have your child explain the *Focus for Clarity* strategy and tell why it's important to know how to define words.
2. Ask your child to tell you the elements that make up a clear and precise definition (i.e., label or name, category, and distinctive feature).
3. Have your child give you the definition of three new words from science, social studies, or spelling class.
4. If your child completes these activities, please sign below and return this form to school.

Family Member: ______________________________ Date: ____________________

Homework Activity

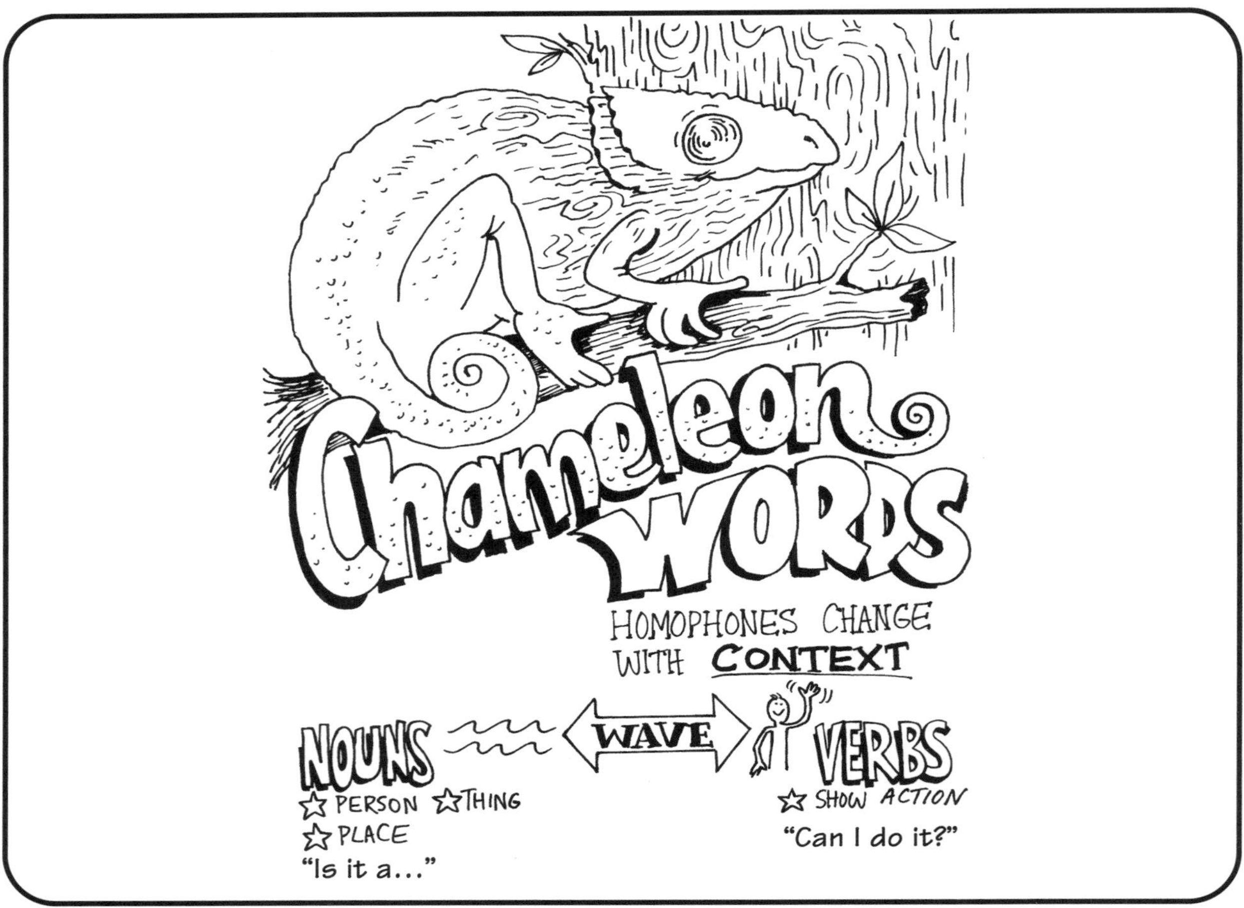

Dear Family,

1. Have your child explain the *Chameleon Words* strategy and tell why it's important to know that some words can have more than one meaning.

2. Look at the sports section of the newspaper or watch the sports portion of the evening news together. Pick three words with multiple meanings to talk about. (Reading the headlines in the sports section of the newspaper will give you lots of ideas.) Have your child tell you the meaning intended in the sports headline and tell you one or more other meanings.

3. If your child completes these activities, please sign below and return this form to school.

Family Member: ______________________________ Date: ____________________

UNIT THREE

GOAL SETTING ACTIVITY FOUR

GOAL

To encourage self-improvement through goal setting

BACKGROUND INFORMATION

The main focus of this lesson is to help students learn the steps for goal setting (i.e., identifying a need, formulating a goal, practicing the steps to reach the goal, revising a goal as needed, and evaluating progress toward meeting a goal). Rather than expecting students to set goals independently, the goal-setting process is modeled. The communication goal could be directed by you, but the reflection on how the goal might be useful will be individual for each student, since each student's use of the skills will be different. A few example goals for this unit are:

1. Improve story knowledge;
2. Understand the key story elements; and
3. Understand and tell stories better.

OBJECTIVES

1. Evaluate progress on achieving previously set goals.
2. Tell how previous goals were met.
3. Write a new goal.

MATERIALS

1. *My Goals #4* (See page 208; duplicate one per student.)
2. *My Goals #3* (Completed in *Goal Setting Activity Three)*
3. Chalkboard and chalk

INTRODUCTION

Tie-in to Prior Learning

Remind students that they had identified specific skills that would strengthen their communication, especially word power (e.g., using synonyms to make ideas more interesting, using one-word antonyms, identifying the patterns that form analogies, showing how words can have more than one meaning, and giving clear, precise definitions).

Focus/Relevancy

1. Explain to students that they will be evaluating their progress on achieving previous goals and will write new goals to achieve. Say to them,

   When we evaluate our work, we are deciding if we have done our best work or a good job. We can evaluate our progress by telling ways we can use our skills at school, at home, and in the community. In our next lessons, we will be using the strategies we have been learning to become better at telling and writing stories.

2. Remind students that learning is easier when goals are set and there is a plan for practicing. Setting goals can help students achieve many different skills in school, at home, and someday at a job. Discuss how it feels to accomplish something that was difficult.

LESSON ACTIVITIES

1. Give each student a copy of *My Goals #4* and their completed *My Goals #3.* Have students evaluate how their word power has improved and have them give examples (e.g., "I can give clearer, more interesting descriptions," "I understand and use words that can have more than one meaning when my friends and I are telling riddles"). Ask students to complete the first half of *My Goals #4.* Have them check whether they achieved their goals or whether they need to revise their goals. Remind students that they will want to continue to practice each achieved goal while targeting another for improvement.

2. Point out the "My new goal is" sentence on the goal sheet. To prompt the discussion of the new goal, ask students if they still remember the very first strategy they learned. Ask a student to tell the components of the *Give Me Five* strategy for listening. Discuss listening actively when evaluating information from stories or textbooks. Relate the idea of movie critics who give movies a thumbs-up or thumbs-down rating depending upon how much they liked the movie. Discuss how the critics might make their decisions. To be an informed evaluator, the student needs to know the essential parts of a story. These parts are also referred to as *story grammar* or *story knowledge.* To tell a logical and clear story, the story grammar parts must be included in a story. Tell the students that they will be gaining this story knowledge so they are better evaluators and creators of stories. Write the term *story knowledge* on the board to prompt goal statements for the next set of lessons.

3. Tell students,

    Reading, telling, and writing stories is an excellent way for us to use our communication skills. Whether we are evaluating a story that we have read, or telling or writing a story, we need to be listening actively, describing precisely, and exercising our word power.

4. Guide students through writing story knowledge goals on their goal sheets. Discuss situations where students feel they could apply their story knowledge goals (e.g., at home, when telling about something that happened at school; at school, when writing a story for an English assignment; in the community, when telling a friend about a movie).

CLOSURE

Summarize the lesson, review its relevance for students, and tie it to future learning. Tell students they have set important goals. Remind students that by signing and dating their goal sheets, they are promising to concentrate and work on their goals. On the bottom of the goal sheet is a line for a family member's signature. Have students take the goal sheets home, explain their goals to family members, and return the goal sheets to school for you to sign. When this group of lessons in Unit Three is finished, the students will be able to share their completed *Strategy Guide Booklets* with their families.

My Goals #4

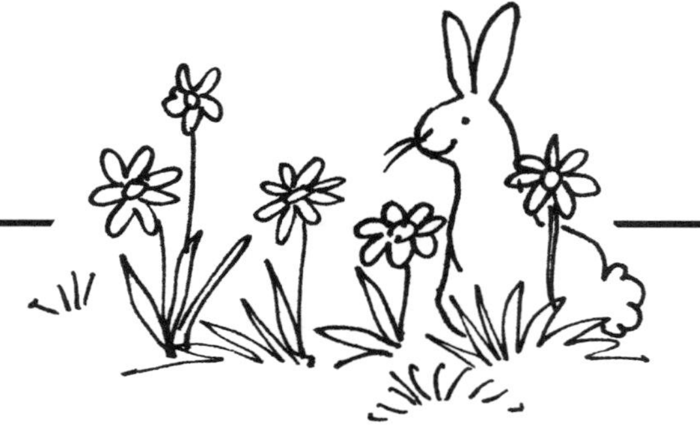

In the last unit, my goals were:

____

____

Now, at home, I ____

____

Now, at school, I ____

____

Now, in the community, I ____

____

☐ I achieved my goal, but will keep practicing it.

☐ I need to revise my goal by ____

____

My new goal is ____

____

At home, I will ____

____

At school, I will ____

____

In the community, I will ____

____

Name: ______________________ Date: ______________

Family Member:______________________ Date: ______________

Teacher: ______________________ Date: ______________

STORY RECIPE: STORY KNOWLEDGE (PART I)

GOAL

To improve story knowledge

BACKGROUND INFORMATION

The main focus of the *Story Recipe* strategy is to improve students' overall narrative language skills by introducing the essential story grammar components and helping students use these components to create their own stories. Before students can be expected to tell, retell, or write clear and logical stories, they must first be able to identify story grammar elements. These are the elements that help a story flow. They are referred to as the *key ingredients* in the next two lessons. Many variations of story grammar elements exist but the elements used in the *Story Recipe* strategy are: setting (including time, place, and characters), problem, solution, and outcome.

OBJECTIVES

1. Identify story grammar components in a story (i.e., setting [including time, place, and characters], problem, solution, and outcome).
2. Identify story grammar components in a reading activity.

MATERIALS

1. *Aunt Isabel Tells a Good One* (1992) by Kate Duke (If desired, substitute another book. This book was selected because it provides a "recipe" for telling or writing stories. It creatively provides a step-by-step process for including all the essential story components in an entertaining format.)
2. *Story Recipe* graphic (See page 212; duplicate and enlarge the graphic, color it, mount it onto poster board, and laminate it for durability, if desired.)
3. Chalkboard and chalk
4. *Story Strip Phrases* (See pages 213–215; duplicate onto heavy stock paper and cut apart; create one set of strips per pair of students.)

INTRODUCTION

Tie-in to Prior Learning

Remind the students of the goals that were set in the last lesson. Relate the idea of having come "full circle" in using all of the communication skills they have learned and now being able to understand, enjoy, and write better stories.

Focus/Relevancy

1. Begin by asking students to name their favorite stories and movies. Have them be specific about why they chose the specific story or movie. Are their choices comedies, adventures, mysteries, etc.? Talk about what students think makes a story good.

2. Address the idea that stories are told every day. Have students brainstorm ideas (e.g., telling events from school or telling what happened while spending the night with a friend). If the speaker knows the story parts of a story, he or she will be better at telling about personal events, retelling movies seen, writing letters, or making up original stories. Tell students,

   We're going to read Aunt Isabel Tells a Good One *by Kate Duke. Let's see if we can figure out what makes this a good story.*

LESSON ACTIVITIES

1. Before reading the story, highlight the literary components (see page 12). Discuss the author and illustrator. In addition, discuss the following:

   - Vocabulary—Define *villains, weeping, panic, odious, lurk, rampage, puny, scurry,* and *screech.*

2. Begin to read the story. While reading, point out the following literary highlights:

   - Vocabulary—Stop at the part in the story when it mentions needing to have "just the right ingredients." Discuss the meaning of the word *ingredients,* and ask what the students think of when they hear that word. Compare telling or writing a story to following a recipe. Ask the students what would happen if, when baking a cake, they left out the sugar. Discuss and relate this to leaving out an essential story ingredient. Discuss the possible results (e.g., the story may not make sense or the story might be dull, as Aunt Isabel said).

   - Story grammar elements—As the key ingredients are mentioned, stop and ask what is needed for the story. List the words on the board: *setting (when, where, who), problem, solution,* and *outcome.*

   - Missing elements—Read up to the part of the story where Bad Egg Bat knocks himself out by hitting his head. Discuss whether this is a good place for the story to end. Is it known what happens to Prince Augustus and Lady Nell or the King and Queen? Does the story need something more? Ask if there are any unanswered questions.

3. After reading the story, point out the following literary highlights:

   - Story elements—Have students answer when, where, who questions about the story. Display the *Story Recipe* poster. Talk about the different ingredients that were mentioned. Discuss the use of additional ingredients (e.g., danger, romance, action) that made the story more enjoyable and exciting.
   - Multiple meaning words—Define *dull, mouth of the cave, bat, racket, dash,* and *hide.*
   - Synonyms and antonyms—Have students identify synonyms and antonyms within the story such as *dark, gloomy, cheerful, sunny, clever, generous, weep, foolish, wise, trail, forest, snarls, dash, courage,* and *dawn.*

4. Pair students. Give each pair a set of *Story Strip Phrases,* which have story elements written on them. Have students practice identifying the story ingredients by reading a strip and deciding which story ingredient is being described. Have each pair share their decisions with the large group.

CLOSURE

Summarize the lesson, review its relevance to students, and tie it to future learning. Explain that the students will have an opportunity to use the story recipe to create their own stories in the next lesson.

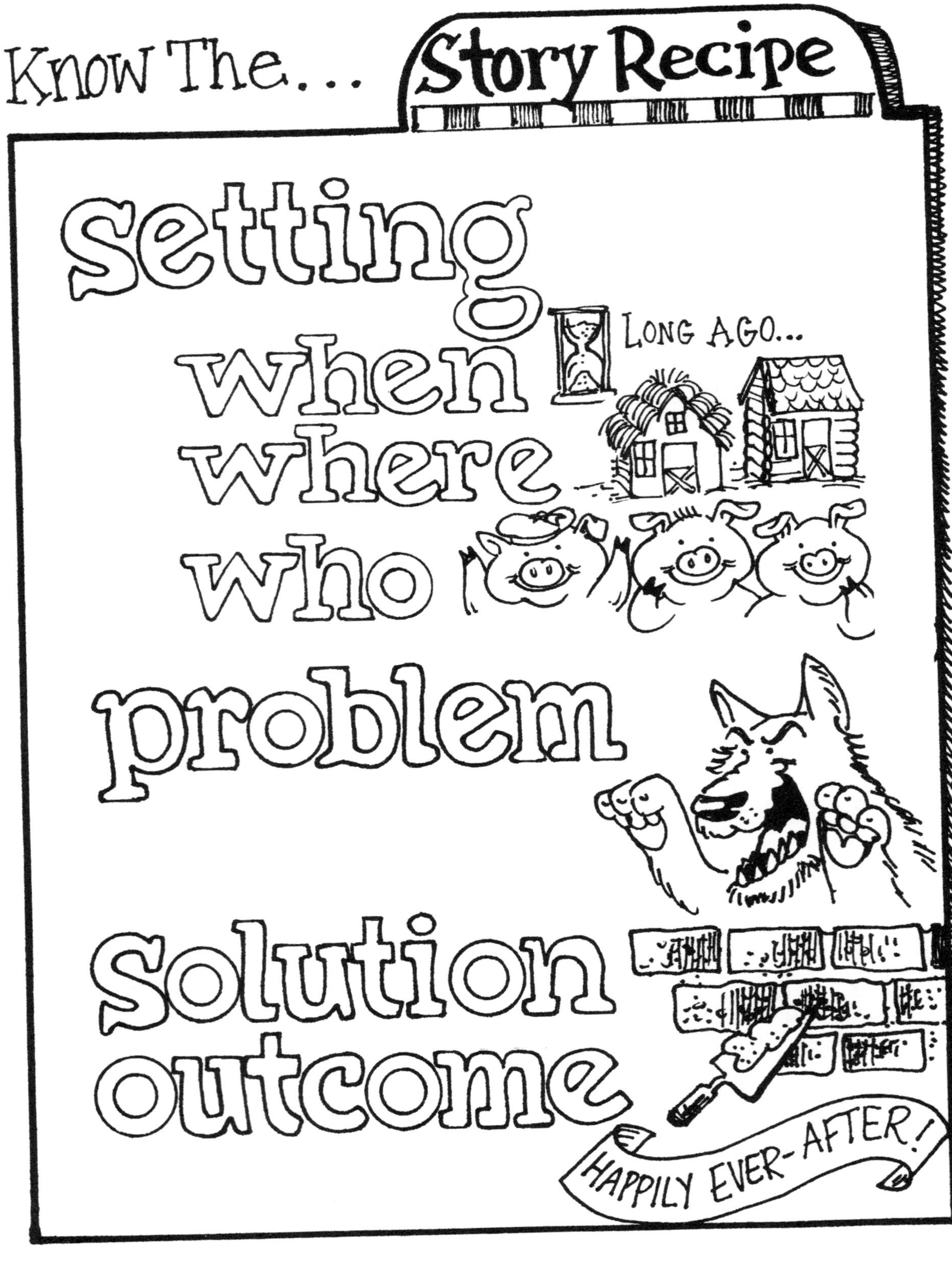

Know The...
Story Recipe
setting
when
LONG AGO...
where
who
problem
solution
outcome
HAPPILY EVER-AFTER!

Story Strip Phrases

a little boy

a hot, steamy jungle

He fell into a muddy river.

climbed onto an alligator and rode to shore

10 noisy monkeys

The lion chased the little boy up the tree.

The boy grabbed a rope and swung out of the monster's reach.

the elephant

the lion

The boy found his parents and they were so happy.

and he was never seen again

Gretchen the cocker spaniel

She was afraid of crawling into his small, dark doghouse.

The duck was afraid of the water.

He got a life preserver to wear.

The lion got ear muffs to protect him from the noise.

He turned on his night-light.

He wanted to make up all the rules and his friends did not like that.

forest, beach, night, city

winter, home, playground

day, country

The friends argued about the game.

The girl enjoyed her trip and looked forward to going again.

I decided to draw my own picture.

She ate a poisoned apple, which made her fall asleep.

She woke up when the prince gave her a kiss.

They lived in a beautiful little house in the woods.

They lived happily ever after in the strong house made of bricks.

The girl had nothing suitable to wear to the ball so she would have to stay home.

The fairy godmother turned her raggedy clothes into a beautiful gown.

They learned to never leave their door unlocked when they took a walk in the woods.

The third brother built his house out of bricks rather than hay or sticks.

STORY RECIPE: STORY KNOWLEDGE (PART II)

GOAL

To improve story knowledge

BACKGROUND INFORMATION

The main focus of the *Story Recipe* strategy is to improve students' overall narrative language skills by introducing the essential story grammar components and helping students use these components to create their own stories. Before students can be expected to tell, retell, or write clear and logical stories, they must first be able to identify story grammar elements. These are the elements that help a story flow. They are referred to as the *key ingredients* in this lesson. Many variations of story grammar elements exist but the elements used in the *Story Recipe* strategy are: setting (including time, place, and characters), problem, solution, and outcome.

OBJECTIVES

1. Identify story grammar components in a story (i.e., setting [including time, place, and characters], problem, solution, and outcome).
2. Use story grammar components in writing activities.

MATERIALS

1. *Story Recipe* poster (Created earlier)
2. *Aunt Isabel Tells a Good One Sequel* (See page 218; duplicate one per student.)

INTRODUCTION

Tie-in to Prior Learning

Refer students to the *Story Recipe* poster and review what the students remember about the essential story ingredients: setting, problem, solution, and outcome.

Focus/Relevancy

1. Ask students if they are familiar with the word *sequel*. If students are unsure, refer to a recent movie that has had a sequel, then see if they can guess what *sequel* means. Relate the idea of a sequel to the Aunt Isabel story. Ask how the story ended. Have students predict what could happen next. Explain that the author predicted what might happen in a future story. Ask students to tell what they would like to happen.

2. Discuss that in school and outside of the classroom, students may be asked to tell, retell, or write stories or accounts of events. Practicing the story recipe will strengthen their skills.

LESSON ACTIVITIES

1. Explain to students that in a sequel, the author adds fresh ingredients to the story (or an element of the story) by changing the setting, presenting a new problem, introducing new characters, etc. while maintaining a connection to the original story. Tell them,

   We're going to be authors of our own sequel to the Aunt Isabel Tells a Good One *story. Since we are the authors and know that there needs to be a connection to the original story, let's think about what might happen next.* (Point to "when" on the poster.) *Should our sequel take place in the present, past, or future?* (Point to "who.") *Will Lady Nell be a grandmother or will the story be about Lady Nell and Prince Augustus's children? Is it far into the future when their great grandchildren live in a space station? Does it take place in the past when their method of transportation would be a horse and carriage? Does our sequel pick up right where the original story left off? You, as the author, get to decide!*

2. Continue giving examples for substituting, combining, adding, modifying, or changing the setting, problem, solution, and/or outcome. Model telling a short sequel with at least one sentence for each story grammar component. Emphasize that if students can tell the sequel, they can also write it.

3. Distribute *Aunt Isabel Tells a Good One Sequel* activity page. Have students write at least one complete sentence for each of the story ingredients: setting (including when, where, and who), problem, solution, and outcome. Stress that with these sentences they will have the basic components for a new story. Briefly discuss information that adds flavor to a story (e.g., mystery, humor, romance, adventure).

4. Allow time for students to write and then share their sequel ideas with each other.

CLOSURE

Summarize the lesson, review its relevance to students, and tie it to future learning. The students will be using their story knowledge to discover the main idea in the *Tell the Biggest Eggs* and *Follow the Detail Trail* lessons.

Aunt Isabel Tells a Good One Sequel

Name: ______________________ Date: ____________

My ideas are:

Setting (including when, where, and who): ______________________

____

____

____

Problem: ______________________

____

____

____

Solution: ______________________

____

____

____

Outcome: ______________________

____

____

____

STORY RECIPE FOLLOW-UP ACTIVITIES

GOAL

To reinforce and review the *Story Recipe* strategy

BACKGROUND INFORMATION

The main focus of this lesson is to review the previous strategy. The strategy guide review pages will be compiled with similar pages into a booklet. This booklet, along with a vacation calendar, provides a means of practicing with family members and reinforcing skills throughout a school break. Although some educators may choose to do the strategy guide pages and homework activities at the end of each lesson, others prefer delayed reinforcement to strengthen knowledge of strategies, concepts, and vocabulary covered within the lessons. Using a small representation of the strategy poster, the strategy guide pages include the specific vocabulary from the lessons. An application component is provided on the second page of the strategy guide. Students may do reflective writing about how the strategy is or can be useful to them.

OBJECTIVES

1. Tell and write the major components of the *Story Recipe* strategy.
2. Reflect and write about how the strategy will help at home, at school, and in the community.
3. Share strategy information with family members and complete the application activities.

MATERIALS

1. *Story Recipe* poster (Created earlier)
2. *Story Recipe Strategy Guide* (See pages 221–222; duplicate one per student.)
3. *Story Recipe Homework Activity* (See page 223; duplicate one per student.)

INTRODUCTION

Tie-in to Prior Learning

Refer students to *Goal Setting Activity Four* (see pages 205–207) and their completed goal sheets. Point out that they have learned one more strategy that will help them improve and move toward achieving their goals. Display the poster and review the *Story Recipe* strategy.

Focus/Relevancy

Review the importance of the *Strategy Guide Booklet* which will be a collection of the student's guide pages for each strategy learned. The booklet will help them become better communicators by helping them remember all the strategies they will be learning. Explain to students that the new pages will be added as new strategies are learned and remind them that the booklet of strategies will be theirs to keep.

LESSON ACTIVITIES

1. Distribute the *Story Recipe Strategy Guide* pages. Students should demonstrate they know the strategy by completing the page with their ingredients for a story. Refer to the poster and have it displayed for the students. Challenge students to expand their ideas into a complete story on another sheet of paper. Keep this story in the students' portfolios.

2. On the second page of the strategy guide, have students write how this particular strategy has helped them or will help them at school, at home, or in the community. Brainstorm ideas (e.g., "When I tell a story about something that has happened to me, I will include important elements so people listening will understand my story," "I told my cousin about the movie *Beauty and the Beast.* I think I got all the parts in because she didn't ask me a lot of questions").

3. Hand out the *Story Recipe Homework Activity* page and discuss it. Reinforce the importance of sharing this information with family members, and the ease and fun of doing these assignments. They will only take a few minutes to complete, but students can impress their family with what they have learned! Have a reward system established to encourage students to bring their homework activity page back to school signed by a family member.

CLOSURE

Summarize the lesson, review its relevance to students, and tie it to future learning. Discuss the objectives that were completed in this review (i.e., the students can tell and write the ingredients in a story; they can tell how they will use the *Story Recipe* strategy; they know the strategy well enough to share it with their family members).

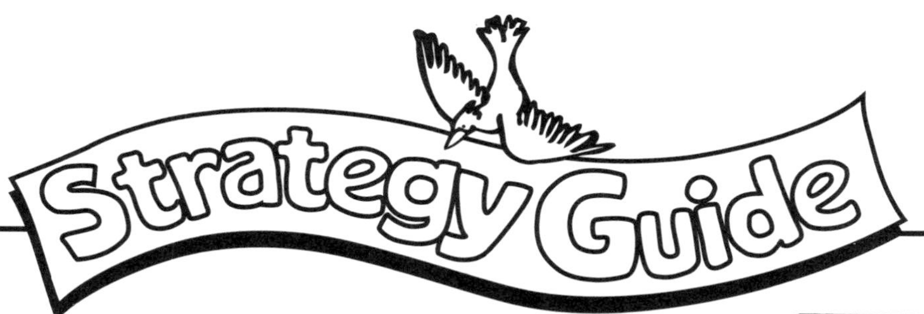

Story Recipe: Story Knowledge

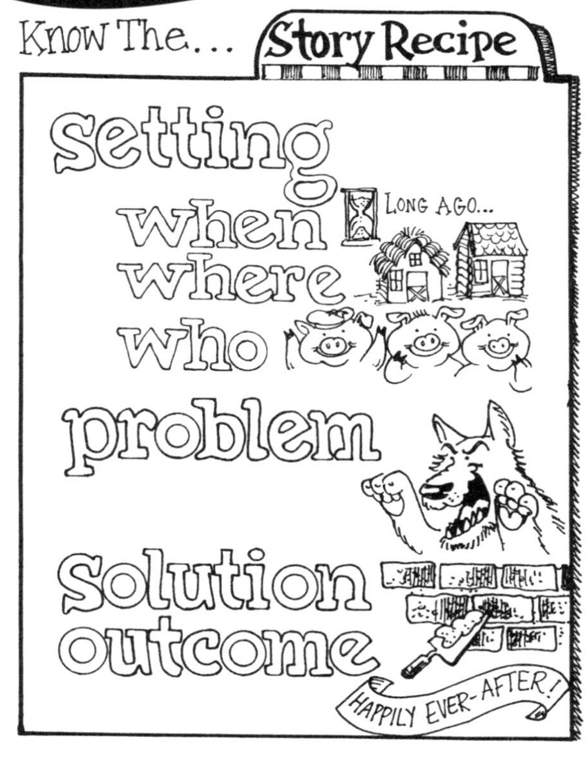

Think of a story, something that happened to you, to your friend, or to your pet. Tell the ingredients.

Setting (when, where, and who):

____

____

____

____

Problem: ________________________

____

____

Solution: ____

____

____

Outcome: ____

____

____

Story Recipe: Story Knowledge

Name: ______________________________ Date: ______________

Directions: Write a sentence about how you have used or will use the strategy in each place.

At home, I ____

____

____

____

____

____

At school, I ____

____

____

____

____

____

In my community, I ____

____

____

____

____

____

Homework Activity

Know The...
Story Recipe
setting
when
LONG AGO...
where
who
problem
solution
outcome
HAPPILY EVER-AFTER!

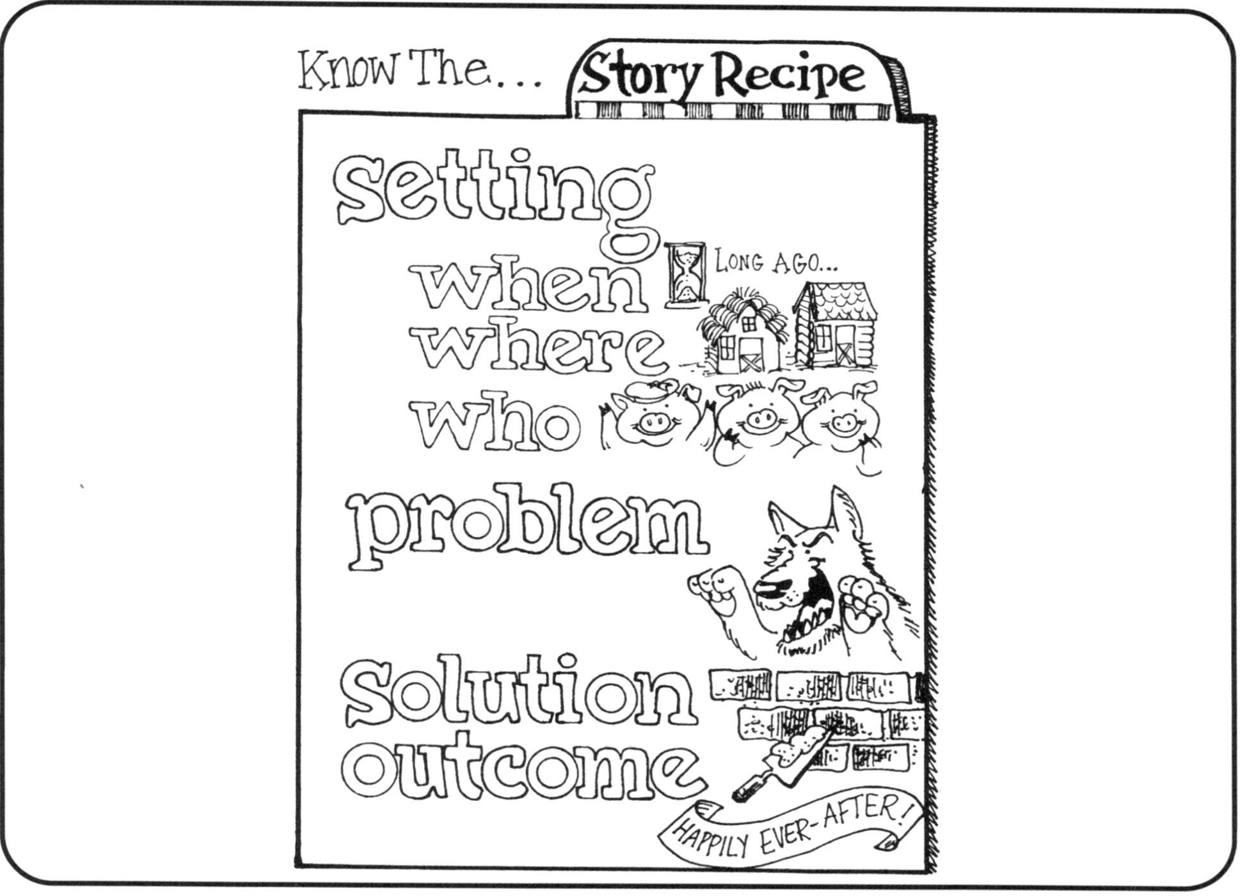

Dear Family,

1. Have your child explain the *Story Recipe* strategy and why it's important to use when telling or writing a story.
2. Ask your child to tell a funny story about something that happened at school. Make sure he or she has included all the story ingredients.
3. Read a story together. After reading the story, ask your child to retell it. Be sure all the story ingredients are included.
4. If your child completes these activities, please sign below and return this form to school.

Family Member: ______________________________ Date: ______________

TELL THE BIGGEST EGGS: MAIN IDEA

GOAL

To improve story knowledge

BACKGROUND INFORMATION

The main focus of the next three lessons is to improve the students' overall story knowledge by helping them learn to summarize the main idea of stories and identify cause and effect relationships within a story. (Before students can be expected to tell the main idea of a story, they will need to be able to identify the story grammar elements.) For the *Tell the Biggest Eggs* strategy, students will summarize the main idea by telling the characters and the most important problem or event in one or two sentences. This is referred to as *Tell the biggest eggs, don't give away all the eggs!*

OBJECTIVES

1. Give the main idea of a story in a one- or two-sentence summary.
2. Summarize the main idea by telling the main character(s) and primary problem or event.

MATERIALS

1. *Tell the Biggest Eggs* graphic (See page 227; duplicate and enlarge the graphic, color it, mount it onto poster board, and laminate it for durability, if desired.)
2. A small grocery bag
3. Seven plastic eggs (Two large and five smaller eggs; see step 1.)
4. *Story Grammar Strips* (See page 228; prepare two sets of strips as described in step 1 of the *Lesson Activities*.)
5. Tape
6. A straw or wire basket to hold the eggs
7. *No Moon, No Milk!* (1993) by Chris Babcock (If desired, substitute another book. *No Moon, No Milk!* was chosen because it has a recognizable theme. It mentions many geographical and cultural locations, which provide interest and opportunities for discussion.)
8. *Biggest Eggs: Main Idea* (See page 229; duplicate one per student.)

INTRODUCTION

Tie-in to Prior Learning

Review the story ingredients for the *Story Recipe* strategy. Provide feedback on the story sequel that the students wrote in the *Story Recipe (Part II)* lesson.

Focus/Relevancy

1. Tell the class that this lesson will be about main ideas. Ask students what a main idea is. Choose a student to give the main idea from *Aunt Isabel Tells a Good One,* or from any familiar story. Respond to the student's summary. If the student gives too many details or tells the whole story, explain that when summarizing the main idea, only certain parts of the story are told. If the student gives a concise summary, emphasize that he or she gave only specific parts of the story to summarize.

2. Stress that finding and telling the main idea is an important skill. Many activities require students to listen to or read a paragraph or story and tell the most important information. In addition, when telling about an enjoyable book or movie, the speaker will want to tell the main idea to grab the listener's interest.

LESSON ACTIVITIES

1. Before this lesson, create a set of eggs as follows: label the two larger eggs as "Main Characters" and "Main Problem or Event"; label the smaller eggs "Details," "Setting (when)," "Setting (where)," "Solution," and "Outcome." Enlarge and duplicate one set of *Story Grammar Strips* onto heavy stock paper; cut apart to form strips. Duplicate and decrease in size another set of *Story Grammar Strips;* cut the strips apart and place them in the eggs, sorting by story ingredient.

2. Hold up the bag of eggs for all to see. Remove the eggs from the bag and ask students what the labels represent. Elicit the story ingredient concept. Have different students come up one at a time to read the egg labels, open the egg, and read the *Story Grammar Strip* inside. As the student reads the strip, tape the larger corresponding *Story Grammar Strip* on a wall or bulletin board for easier reading. After each small strip is read, put it back inside the egg and place the egg in the basket.

3. To illustrate a main idea, read a detail from the posted *Story Grammar Strips* and ask if it would tell what a story is mainly about (e.g., "Is this story mainly about long, long ago on a dark and stormy night?"). Stress that when students are giving a summary, they must choose the most important information. Show the basket of eggs as a clue. Ask if anyone notices something distinguishing about some of the eggs. Prompt for the identification of the two larger eggs. Have two students read the labels on these eggs and have two other students find the associated *Story Grammar Strips*. Ask the students to move the strips to one side. Using a carrier phrase (e.g., "This story is mainly about ____, who _____..."), model the formulation of a one-sentence summary (e.g., "This story is mainly about a prince and a princess who croak like frogs because an evil queen cast a spell on the...").

4. Show the *Tell the Biggest Eggs* poster. Remind students that a main idea tells the biggest egg; you don't have to cluck out the whole story and give away all the eggs when someone asks you the main idea of a story. Discuss how this strategy will work when summarizing a movie, a story from a book, or even a personal experience (e.g., to tell the main idea of *The Wizard of Oz* you might say, "A girl named Dorothy was caught in a tornado. She got stuck in Oz and didn't know how to get back").

5. Before reading the story *No Moon, No Milk!*, highlight the literary components (see page 12). Discuss the author and illustrator. In addition, discuss the following:

   - Main idea—Ask students to predict the main idea by looking at the cover of the book. Allow several predictions.

6. Read the story. While reading the story, point out the following literary highlights:

   - Vocabulary—Define *quivering, bellowing, stampede, passel of skaters, replica, lunar, restrain, bovine, domesticated,* and *crater.*

7. After reading the story, point out the following literary highlights:

   - Story grammar elements—Review the story's ingredients: the setting (including the characters), the problem, the solution, and the outcome. In addition, identify unimportant details.

   - Figurative language—Discuss the figurative terms *hang ten* and *one small step for cow, one giant leap for cowkind.*

8. Distribute *Biggest Eggs: Main Idea* activity sheets to students. Ask the students what information from *No Moon, No Milk!* should be included in the larger eggs, and then have them write the main characters and main problem on the lines next to the large eggs. Have them fill in setting, solution, outcome, and other details on the lines by the the smaller eggs. Finally, have them write a summary sentence telling the main idea of the story (e.g., "The story is mainly about a cow who will not let the farmer milk her until she gets to go to the moon"). Note that some students will have difficulty writing a complex sentence such as this so a two-sentence summary should be allowed.

CLOSURE

Summarize the lesson, review its relevance to students, and tie it to future learning. Let students share their summary sentences. Apply the *Tell the Biggest Eggs* strategy and the idea of "Not giving away all the eggs" to a story or passage from a classroom activity. Tell students that in the next lesson, they will be learning another strategy to improve their story knowledge: identifying cause and effect in a story. Have students recall being asked to summarize main ideas in other classes.

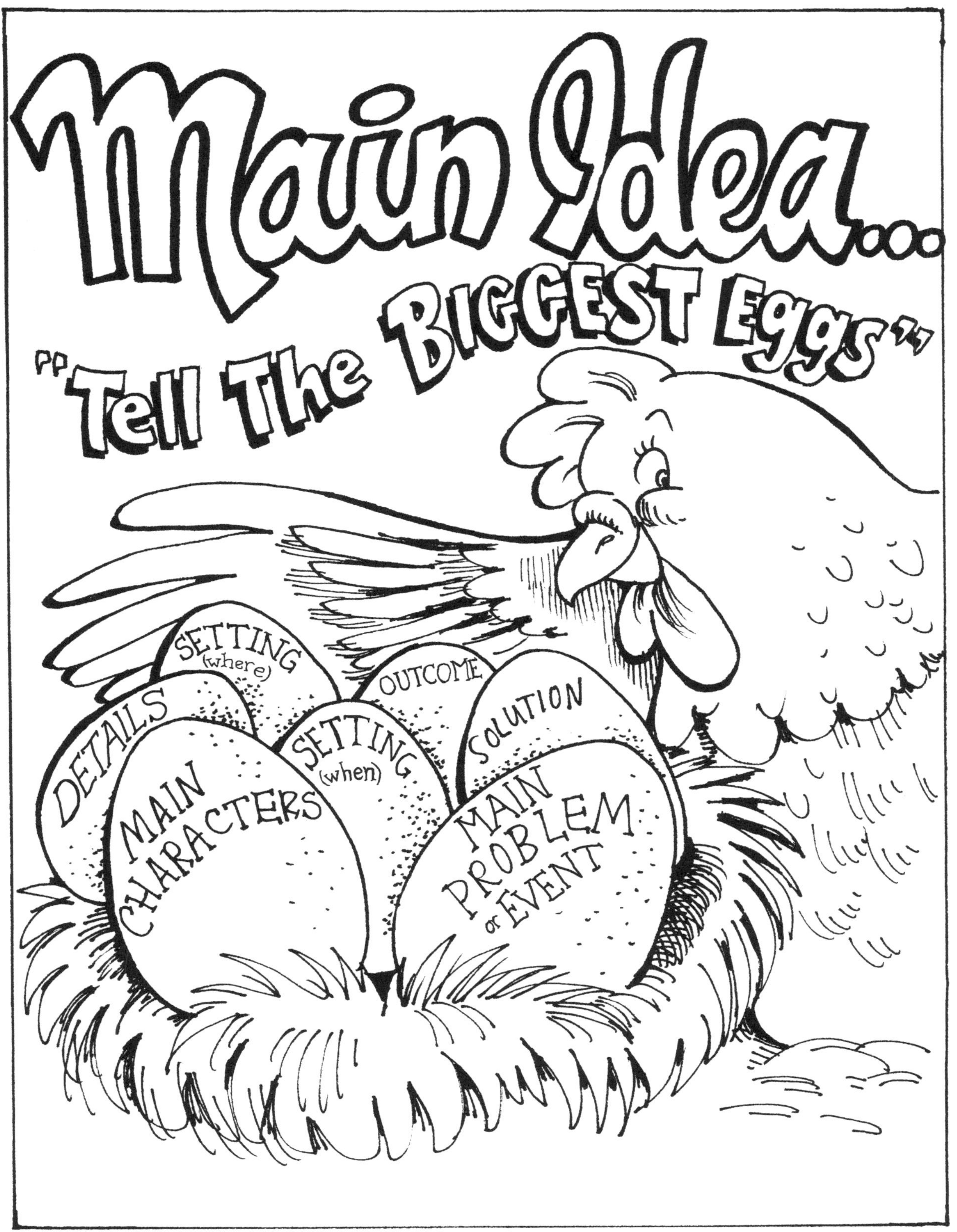
Main Idea...
"Tell The BIGGEST Eggs"
SETTING (where)
OUTCOME
DETAILS
SETTING (when)
SOLUTION
MAIN CHARACTERS
MAIN PROBLEM or EVENT

Story Grammar Strips

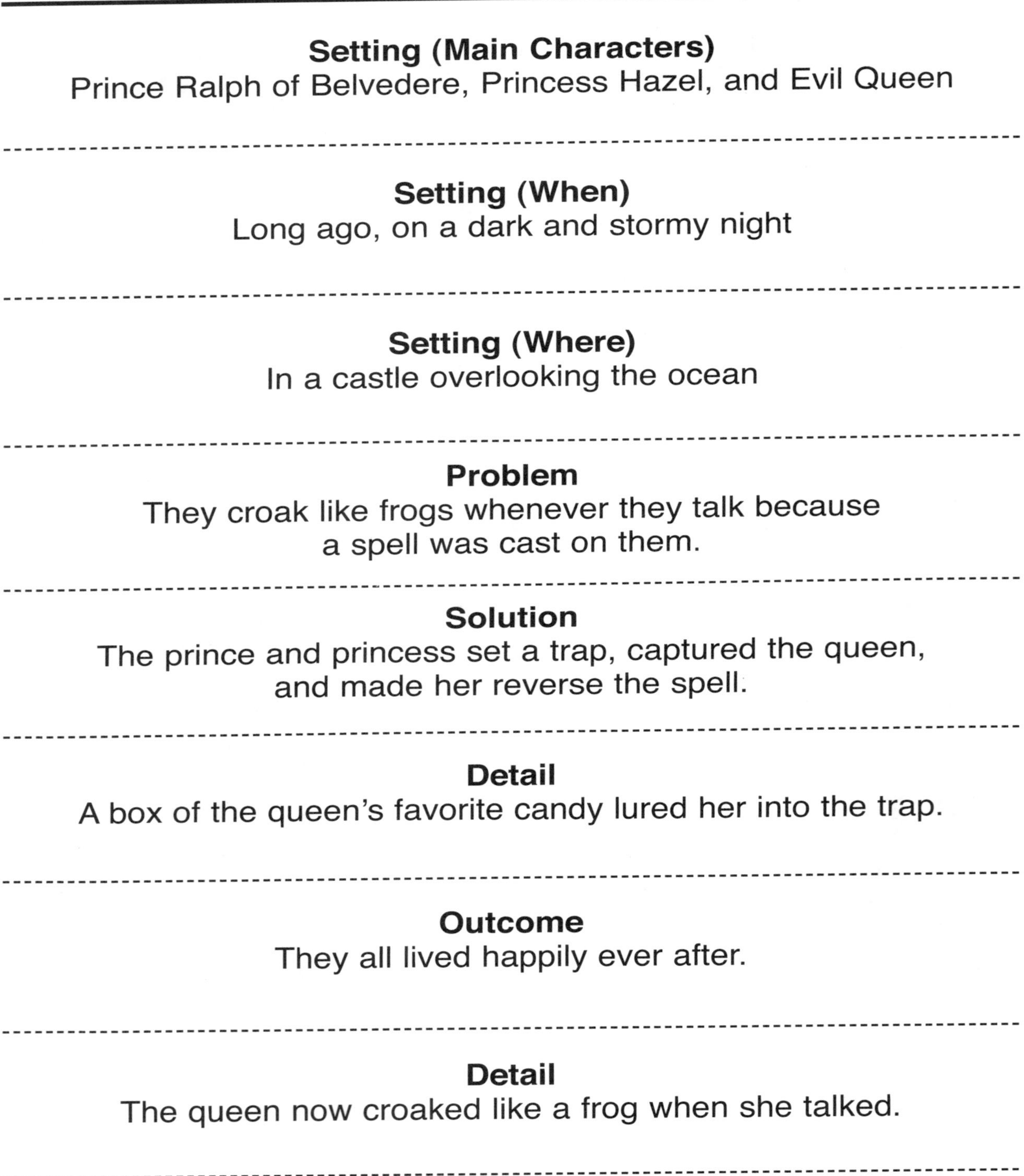

Setting (Main Characters)
Prince Ralph of Belvedere, Princess Hazel, and Evil Queen

Setting (When)
Long ago, on a dark and stormy night

Setting (Where)
In a castle overlooking the ocean

Problem
They croak like frogs whenever they talk because a spell was cast on them.

Solution
The prince and princess set a trap, captured the queen, and made her reverse the spell.

Detail
A box of the queen's favorite candy lured her into the trap.

Outcome
They all lived happily ever after.

Detail
The queen now croaked like a frog when she talked.

Biggest Eggs: Main Idea

Name: ______________________ Date: ______________

Story: ______________________________________

Directions: Write the story ingredients on the lines provided. Then write one or two sentences summarizing the main idea of the story.

Main Characters ______________________________________

____

Main Problem or Event ______________________________________

____

Setting (where) ______________________________________

____

Setting (when) ______________________________________

____

Solution ______________________________________

____

Outcome ______________________________________

____

Details ______________________________________

____

Main Idea Summary: ______________________________________

____

____

FOLLOW THE DETAIL TRAIL: CAUSE AND EFFECT (PART I)

GOAL

To improve story knowledge

BACKGROUND INFORMATION

The main focus of the *Follow the Detail Trail* strategy is to increase the students' overall story knowledge by helping them identify cause and effect relationships within a story. The students will be identifying, answering, and/or asking questions to discover cause and effect relationships and will identify other key words that signal cause and effect.

OBJECTIVES

1. Understand the meaning of *cause* and *effect.*
2. Identify cause and effect relationships within a story.
3. Recognize and use key words that signal cause and effect relationships.

MATERIALS

1. A bag or container with treats (One treat per student)
2. Chalkboard and chalk
3. *A River Ran Wild* (1992) by Lynne Cherry (If desired, substitute another book. This book was chosen because it includes a number of different language concepts and because of its historical content. It creatively traces the effects of industrialization upon a particular river. The story lends itself to discussions about ecology, geography, and responsibility to the world community. It clearly illustrates examples of cause and effect relationships.)
4. *Follow the Detail Trail* graphic (See page 233; duplicate and enlarge the graphic, color it, mount it onto poster board, and laminate it for durability, if desired.)

INTRODUCTION

Tie-in to Prior Learning

Review story knowledge covered up to this point (i.e., story ingredients and main ideas). Students now have the tools to capture a listener's interest by telling the main idea in a story. Discuss that sometimes the listener may want to know more about a story. He or she may ask questions to gather more details (e.g., Why did something happen? What happened when …?).

Focus/Relevancy

1. Show a bag or container filled with some type of treat. After students react excitedly, ask them why they are smiling or excited. Emphasize the word *because* when given in the students' responses. Ask the students why they think they might be receiving a treat. Again emphasize the word *because* in their responses.

2. Enthusiastically tell students that they have just demonstrated a cause and effect relationship. Write the word *why* and the word *effect* beside it in parentheses. Write the word *because* and the word *cause* alongside it in parentheses. Discuss several simple examples of this relationship (e.g., If you turn in an assignment, you will get a grade for it; if you don't eat nutritious food, you will get sick).

3. Ask the students why they were smiling when you held up the container of treats. Below the words *why (effect),* draw a happy face. Under the words *because (cause),* draw the treat that's in the container.

4. Relate cause and effect to problem solving by asking if the students have ever gone into a room and found a toy broken or something spilled on the floor and wondered how these events could have happened. Discuss that people learn to avoid or prevent problems by examining the causes and effects of what happens around them.

LESSON ACTIVITIES

1. Before reading the story, *A River Ran Wild,* highlight the literary components (see page 12). Discuss the author and illustrator. In addition, discuss the following:

   - Main idea—Predict what the story might be about from the cover. Take a few minutes to discuss the cover. Ask the students if they know of another book by this author (e.g., *The Great Kapok Tree).*

2. Tell students that as you read this story, you're going to be asking questions about it. Have them try to recognize a pattern for the kinds of questions you ask. Ask "why" questions throughout the story. Emphasize cause and effect until the students recognize the pattern.

   While reading the story, ask the following questions:

   - Why did the Indians name the river Nashua?
   - Why did the Indians settle by this river?
   - Why do you think the Indians killed only what they needed?

- Why did the settlers "clear" the forests?
- Why did the Indians begin to fight the settlers?
- Why did the Nashua's fish and wildlife begin to get sick?
- Why did the factories dump wastes into the river?
- Why did people and animals start to avoid the river?
- Why did Oweana visit Marion?
- Why were new laws dealing with pollution passed?

3. Ask the students how they answered the "why" questions. Point out that a "why" question needs a "because" answer. When a speaker asks "why," he or she is asking about the cause of an event. When the listener gives a "because" answer, he or she is stating the effect of the event.

4. After reading the story, point out the following literary highlights:

   - Multiple meaning words—Discuss these multiple meaning words as they occurred in the story: *herd/heard, bank, school, settle, dye, power, land.*

   - Vocabulary—Define *migration, quench, generation, nestled, bolts (of cloth), wares, trading post, conquer, pelts, current, dams, pulp, trespass, industrial revolution, fiber, progress, invention, clogged, decomposed, stench, murky, descendent, mourned, cleansed, restore, persuade, fragrant, thatch,* and *vivid.*

   - Figurative language—Define these figurative language terms: *boatload of treasures, bows and arrows were "no match" against gunpowder, towering forest, wars raged, bad smells welled up from the river,* and *the Nashua was slowly dying.*

5. Show the *Follow the Detail Trail* poster. Point out the "because" stepping stone on the detail trail. Discuss the other stepping stones that have cause/effect key words (i.e., conjunctions) written on them.

CLOSURE

Summarize the lesson, review its relevance to students, and tie it to future learning. Ask students to name words that signal an effect and the corresponding words that signal the cause. Have each student tell of one cause and effect situation. Tell the students that in the next lesson they will have an opportunity to practice finding and making their own cause and effect statements.

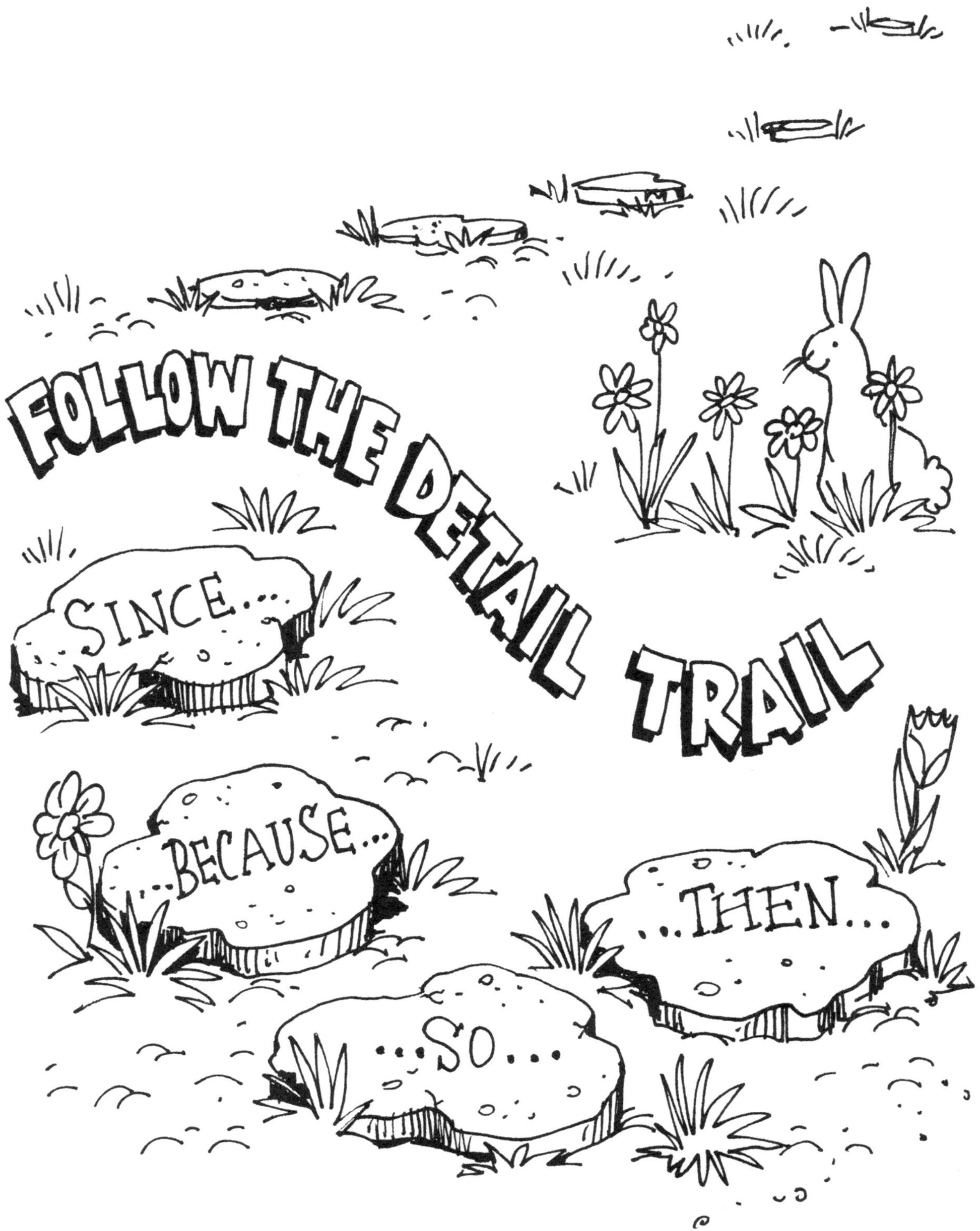
FOLLOW THE DETAIL TRAIL
SINCE...
...BECAUSE...
...THEN...
...SO...

FOLLOW THE DETAIL TRAIL: CAUSE AND EFFECT (PART II)

GOAL

To improve story knowledge

BACKGROUND INFORMATION

The main focus of the *Follow the Detail Trail* strategy is to increase the students' overall story knowledge by helping them identify cause and effect relationships within a story. The students will be identifying, answering, and/or asking questions to discover cause and effect relationships and will identify other key words that signal cause and effect.

OBJECTIVES

1. Understand the meaning of *cause* and *effect.*
2. Identify cause and effect relationships within a story.
3. Recognize and use key words signaling cause and effect relationships.

MATERIALS

1. *Follow the Detail Trail* poster (Created earlier)
2. *Rock Patterns* (See pages 236–237; duplicate the rocks onto gray construction paper [or color them gray] and cut them out.)

INTRODUCTION

Tie-in to Prior Learning

Review the why/effect and because/cause examples that were included in the *Follow the Detail Trail (Part I)* lesson. Review the *Follow the Detail Trail* poster.

Focus/Relevancy

1. Lead students to think about cause and effect in relation to the author of *A River Ran Wild.* Ask students,

   Why do you think Lynne Cherry wrote A River Ran Wild? *She also wrote a book titled* The Great Kapok Tree *which is about saving the rainforest. We may not know for sure, but we can make an educated guess, or infer the reasons this author wrote these books. She seems to be concerned for the environment of the world. When we find causes and effects, we can change how we do things. We can also prevent problems from happening again.*

2. Relate cause and effect to problem solving as the author did in *A River Ran Wild*. Discuss that people learn by discovering the causes of effects around them.

LESSON ACTIVITIES

1. Pass out all 14 paper rocks in random order. Ask the student who has rock #1 to read it for the class and then place it on a bulletin board or tape it to the wall. Explain that this is the effect half of a cause and effect statement. Have students generate a "why" question from this statement (e.g., "Why did the native people build a village along the river bank?"). Ask the group if anyone has the because/cause portion of the statement. Place the *cause* rock on the board next to the *effect* rock once it is identified. This will begin the "detail trail." Continue with rock #2 and so on until the trail is completed. Discuss the *Follow the Detail Trail* poster.

2. Demonstrate other key words (i.e., conjunctions) that signal cause and effect relationships by modeling a *so* statement (e.g., "The native people found a beautiful river, *so* they built a village along its banks"). In this sentence, the word *so* signals an effect. Have students brainstorm other cause and effect conjunctions such as *if/then, since, as a result of,* write them on the board, and give an example of each.

3. As an option to add more challenge, model a cause and effect statement using *because* (e.g., "The river was dirty because garbage was dumped into it"). Write the sentence on the board and challenge students to say it another way by rearranging the words. Give the students the following hint: Look for two big chunks of information to switch. Model the new sentence, "Because the garbage was dumped into the river, it was dirty." Practice with other steps in the detail trail or with other cause and effect statements.

CLOSURE

Summarize the lesson, review its relevance to students, and tie it to future learning. Have students think about how cause and effect relationships in their lives have helped them learn a lesson. Have students look through classroom assignments and identify cause and effect relationships by looking for key words. In the next lesson, students will be completing their *Strategy Guide Booklets* and reviewing these strategies.

Rock Patterns

because
they found a beautiful,
clean river with
sparkling water.
1.
A group of native people
built a village along
this river bank...
2.
The Indians began
to fight the settlers...
3.
Leftover pulp, dye, and
fiber were dumped
into the Nashua River...
because
the settlers cleared
and claimed the land.
4.
The Nashua's fish and
wildlife began to get
sick and die...
because
with the beginning of the industrial
revolution, factories produced much
waste that needed disposal.

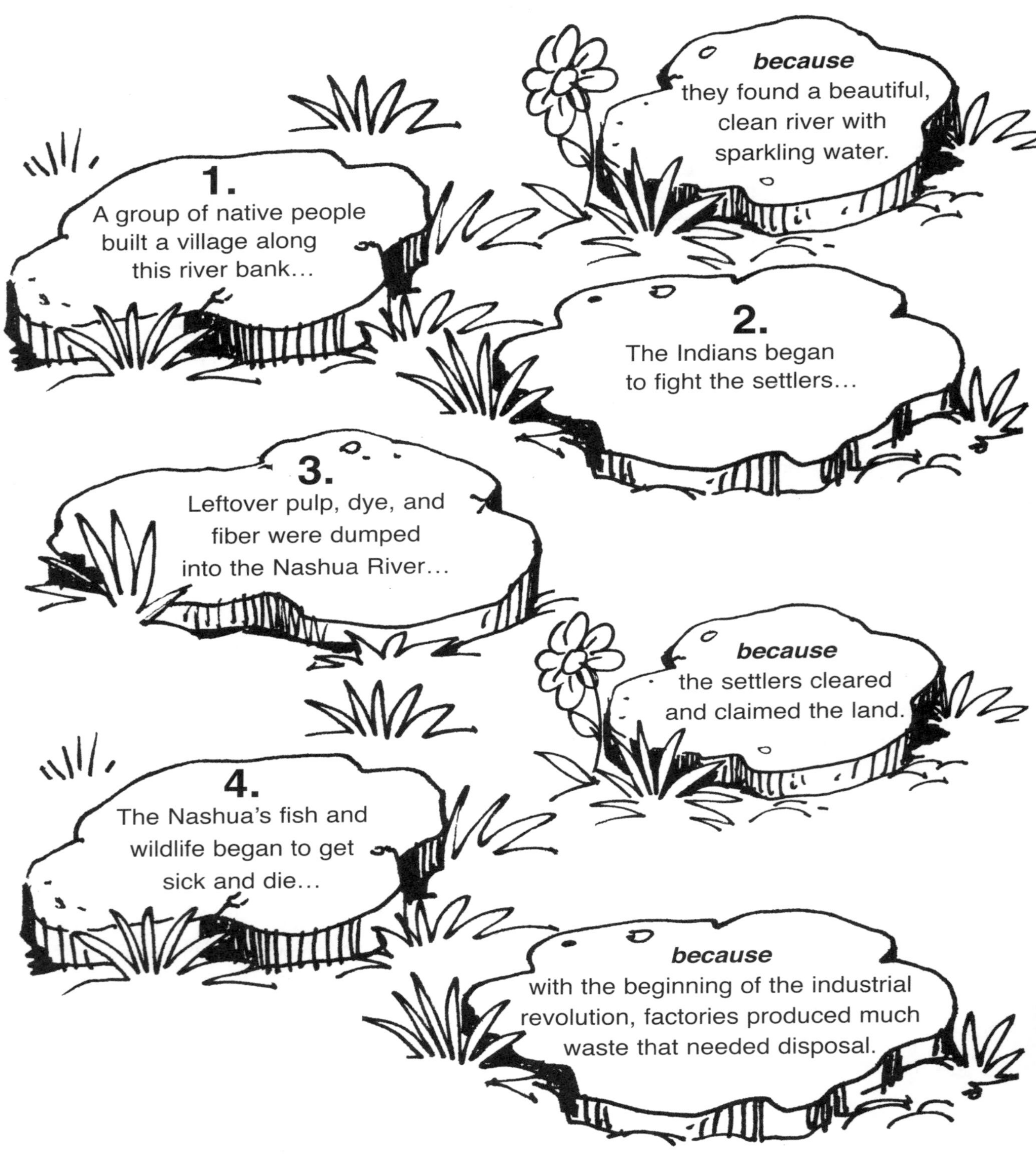

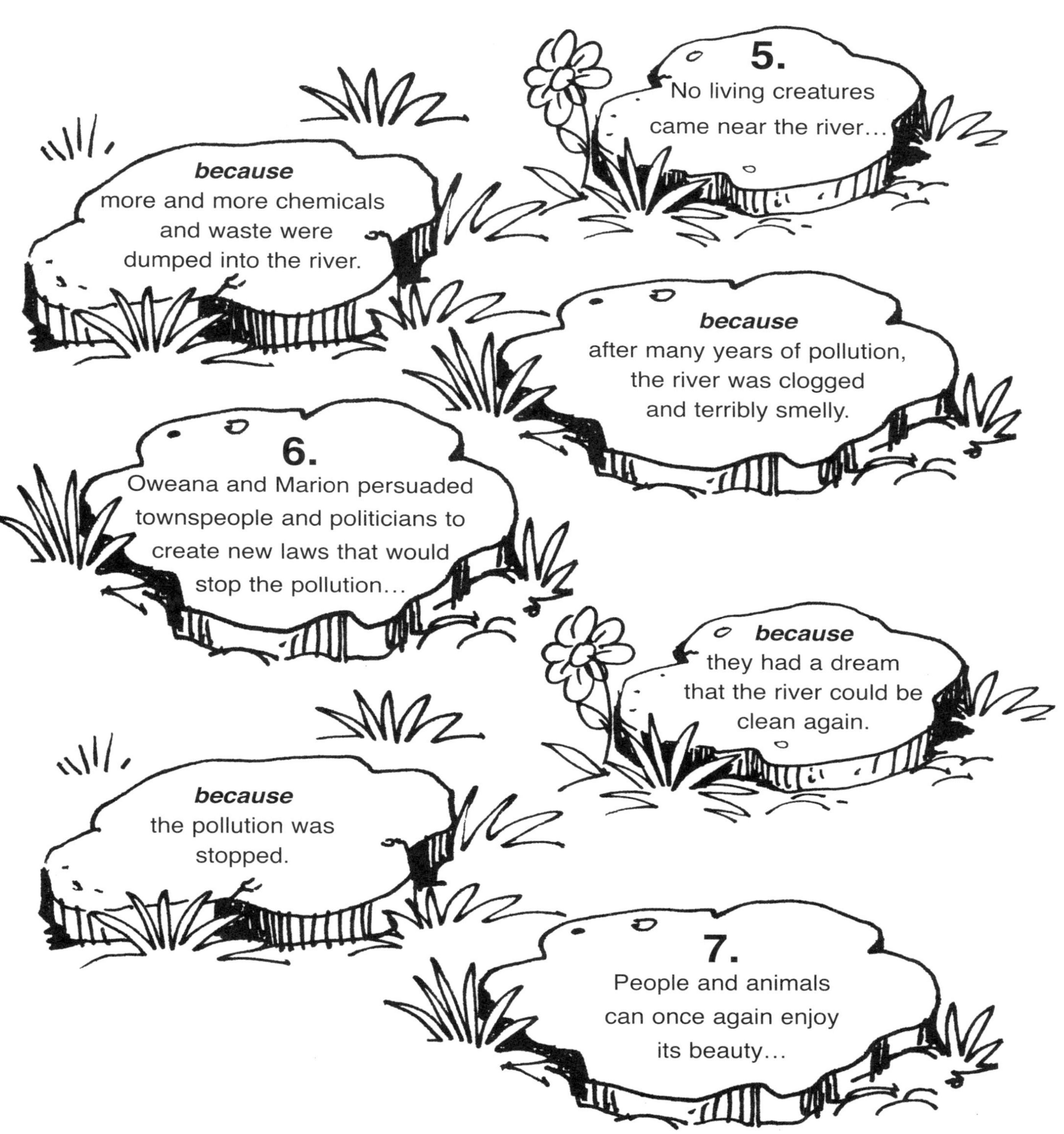
5.
No living creatures
came near the river...
because
more and more chemicals
and waste were
dumped into the river.
because
after many years of pollution,
the river was clogged
and terribly smelly.
6.
Oweana and Marion persuaded
townspeople and politicians to
create new laws that would
stop the pollution...
because
they had a dream
that the river could be
clean again.
because
the pollution was
stopped.
7.
People and animals
can once again enjoy
its beauty...

TELL THE BIGGEST EGGS and FOLLOW THE DETAIL TRAIL FOLLOW-UP ACTIVITIES

GOAL

To reinforce and review *Tell the Biggest Eggs* and *Follow the Detail Trail* strategies

BACKGROUND INFORMATION

The main focus of this lesson is to review the previous two strategies. The strategy guide review pages will be compiled with similar pages into a booklet. This booklet, along with a vacation calendar, provides a means of practicing with family members and reinforcing skills throughout a school break. Although some educators may choose to do the strategy guide pages and homework activities at the end of each lesson, others prefer delayed reinforcement to strengthen knowledge of strategies, concepts, and vocabulary covered within the lessons. Using a small representation of the strategy poster, the strategy guide pages include the specific vocabulary from the lessons. An application component is provided on the second pages of the strategy guides. Students may do reflective writing about how the strategy is or can be useful to them.

OBJECTIVES

1. Tell and write the major components of the *Tell the Biggest Eggs* and *Follow the Detail Trail* strategies.
2. Reflect and write about how the strategies will help at home, at school, and in the community.
3. Share strategy information with family members and complete the application activities.

MATERIALS

1. *Tell the Biggest Eggs* poster (Created earlier)
2. *Follow the Detail Trail* poster (Created earlier)
3. *Tell the Biggest Eggs Strategy Guide* (See pages 240–241; duplicate one per student.)
4. *Follow the Detail Trail Strategy Guide* (See pages 242–243; duplicate one per student.)
5. *Tell the Biggest Eggs Homework Activity* (See page 244; duplicate one per student.)
6. *Follow the Detail Trail Homework Activity* (See page 245; duplicate one per student.)

INTRODUCTION

Tie-in to Prior Learning

Remind the students that they have now learned two more strategies that will help them move toward achieving their goals to improve story knowledge. Display and discuss the posters and strategies for these lessons. Have students tell about each of the strategies in their own words.

Focus/Relevancy

Review the importance of the *Strategy Guide Booklet* which will be a collection of the student's guide pages for each strategy learned. The booklet will help them become better communicators by helping them remember all the strategies they have learned. Remind students that new pages are added as new strategies are learned. Say to them,

> *We're ready to add the very last pages to our* Strategy Guide Booklet *to help remember the important strategies we've learned. I have been looking at all the work you have done so far this year, and now the book is almost complete. We are ready to add the final pages today. Won't your families be amazed at your knowledge about stories and your ability to demonstrate effective communication skills?*

LESSON ACTIVITIES

1. Distribute the *Tell the Biggest Eggs Strategy Guide* pages and the *Follow the Detail Trail Strategy Guide* pages and have students complete them. Students should demonstrate they know the strategies by completing the blank lines. Refer to the posters and have them displayed for the students.
2. On the second page of each strategy guide, have students write how each particular strategy has helped them or will help them at school, at home, or in the community. Brainstorm ideas (e.g., "I had to tell the doctor how I cut my finger. That was cause and effect," "My mom wanted to know what the movie I was watching was about so I just told her the main idea").
3. Hand out the *Tell the Biggest Eggs* and the *Follow the Detail Trail Homework Activity* pages and discuss them. Reinforce the importance of sharing this information with family members, and the ease and fun of doing these assignments. They will only take a few minutes to complete, but students can impress their family with what they have learned! Have a reward system established to encourage students to bring their homework activity pages back to school signed by a family member.
4. Duplicate and assemble each students' *Strategy Guide Booklet* by stapling all the strategy guide pages together. Put one copy in the students' portfolios and keep one for the next lesson.

CLOSURE

Summarize the lesson, review its relevance to students, and tie it to future learning. Discuss the objectives that were completed in this review (i.e., the students can tell and write the *Tell the Biggest Eggs* and *Follow the Detail Trail* strategies; they can tell how they will use the strategies; and they know the strategies well enough to share them with their family members).

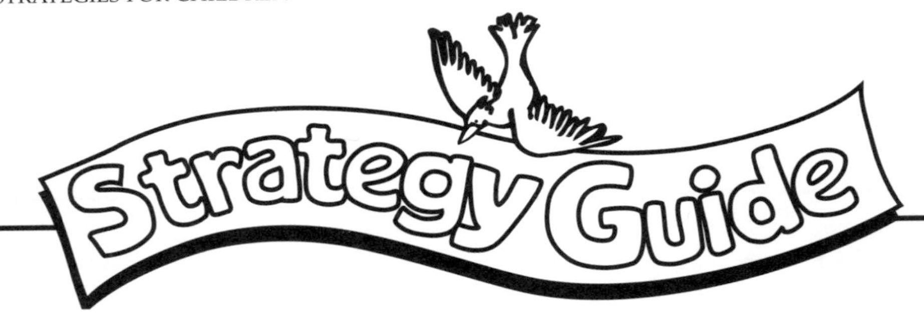

Telling the Main Idea

Practice summarizing the main idea by telling the main characters and main problem or event for a favorite story.

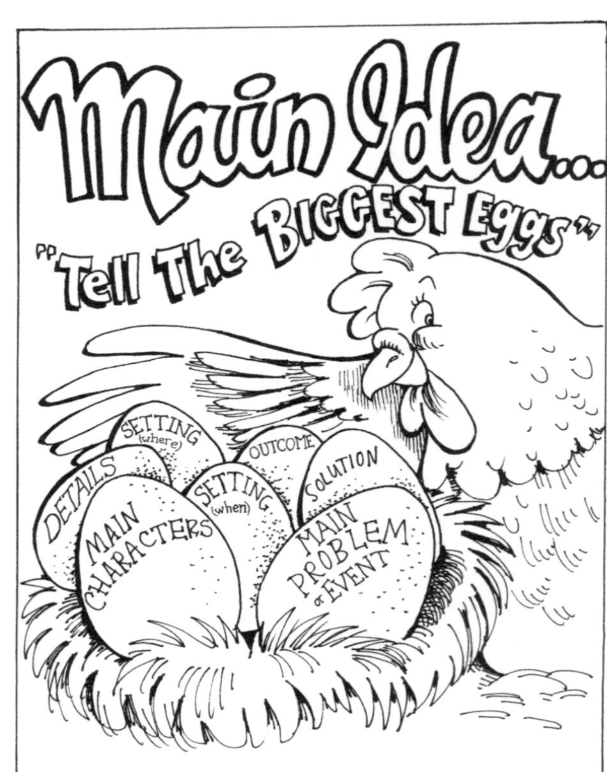

Name of story:

____

____

____

It's mainly about ______________________________

____

____

____

____

who ______________________________

____

______________________________.

Remember: Don't tell all the eggs!

Tell the Biggest Eggs: Main Idea

Name: ______________________________ Date: ______________

Directions: Write a sentence about how you have used or will use the strategy in each place.

At home, I ______________________________

____

____

____

____

____

At school, I ______________________________

____

____

____

____

____

In my community, I ______________________________

____

____

____

____

____

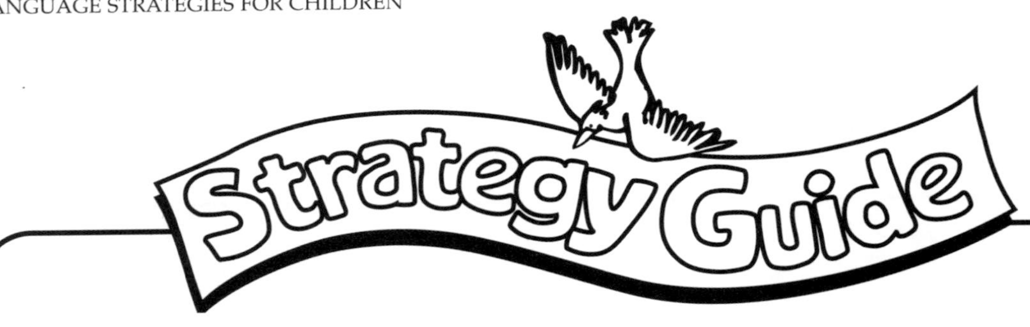

Listen for Cause and Effect

1. Draw a line to match the following *causes* with their *effects.*

cause	effect
no rain	cavities
factories	dry plants
germs	pollution
not brushing	colds

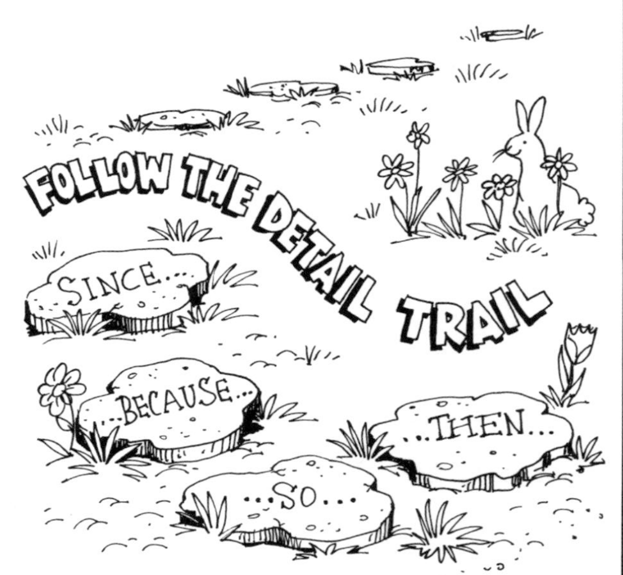

2. Write a complete sentence to explain one of the cause and effect relationships above. Remember to use a cause and effect key word (a conjunction) to join your ideas.

Follow the Detail Trail: Cause and Effect

Name: ______________________________ Date: ______________

Directions: Write a sentence about how you have used or will use the strategy in each place.

At home, I ______________________________

____

____

____

____

____

At school, I ______________________________

____

____

____

____

____

In my community, I ______________________________

____

____

____

____

____

Homework Activity

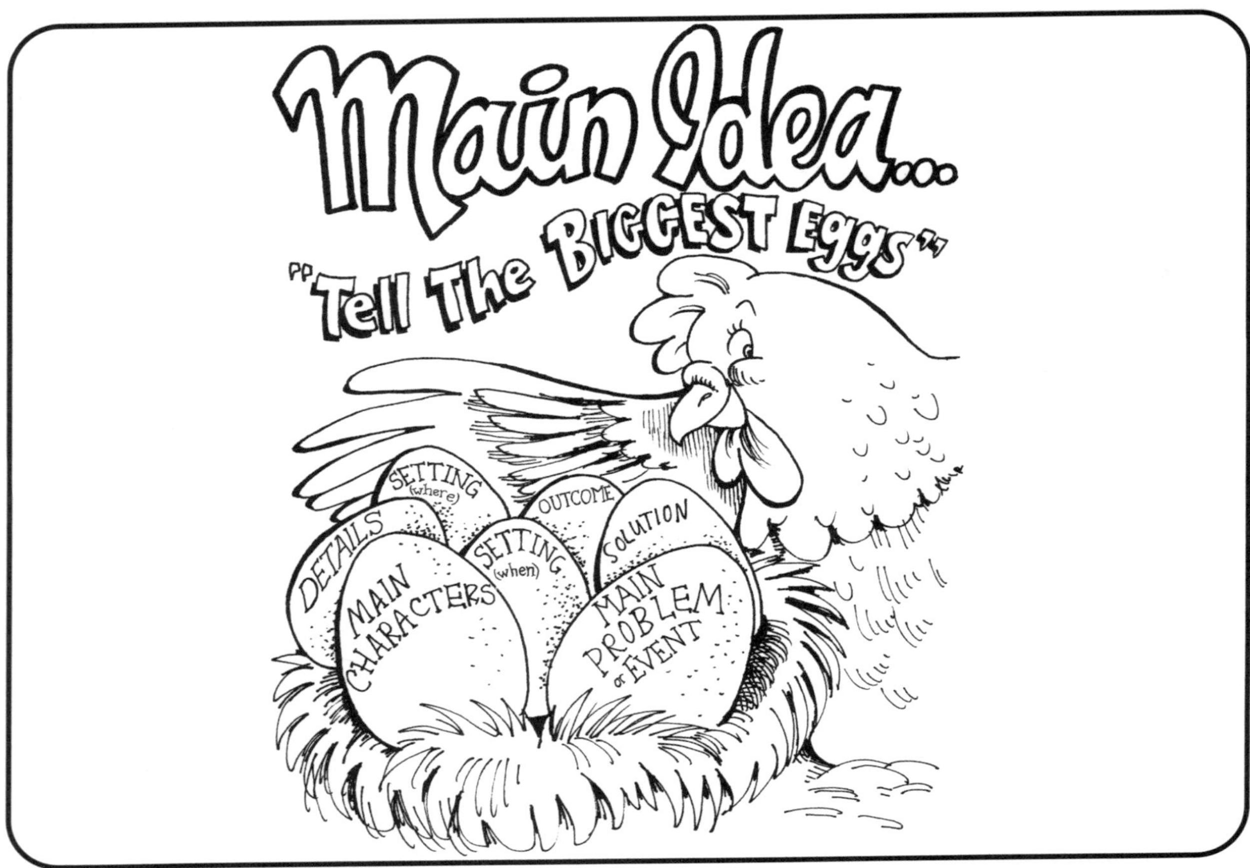

Dear Family,

1. Have your child explain the *Tell the Biggest Eggs* strategy and tell why it's important to know how to summarize main ideas.
2. Help your child practice summarizing main ideas by having him or her tell the main character(s) and main problem or event(s) for:
   a. a favorite book or story
   b. a favorite movie

   Only one or two sentences should be used for the summary.
3. Watch a TV program together and discuss it. Ask your child to summarize the program's main idea.
4. If your child completes these activities, please sign below and return this form to school.

Family Member: ________________________________ Date: ______________________

Homework Activity

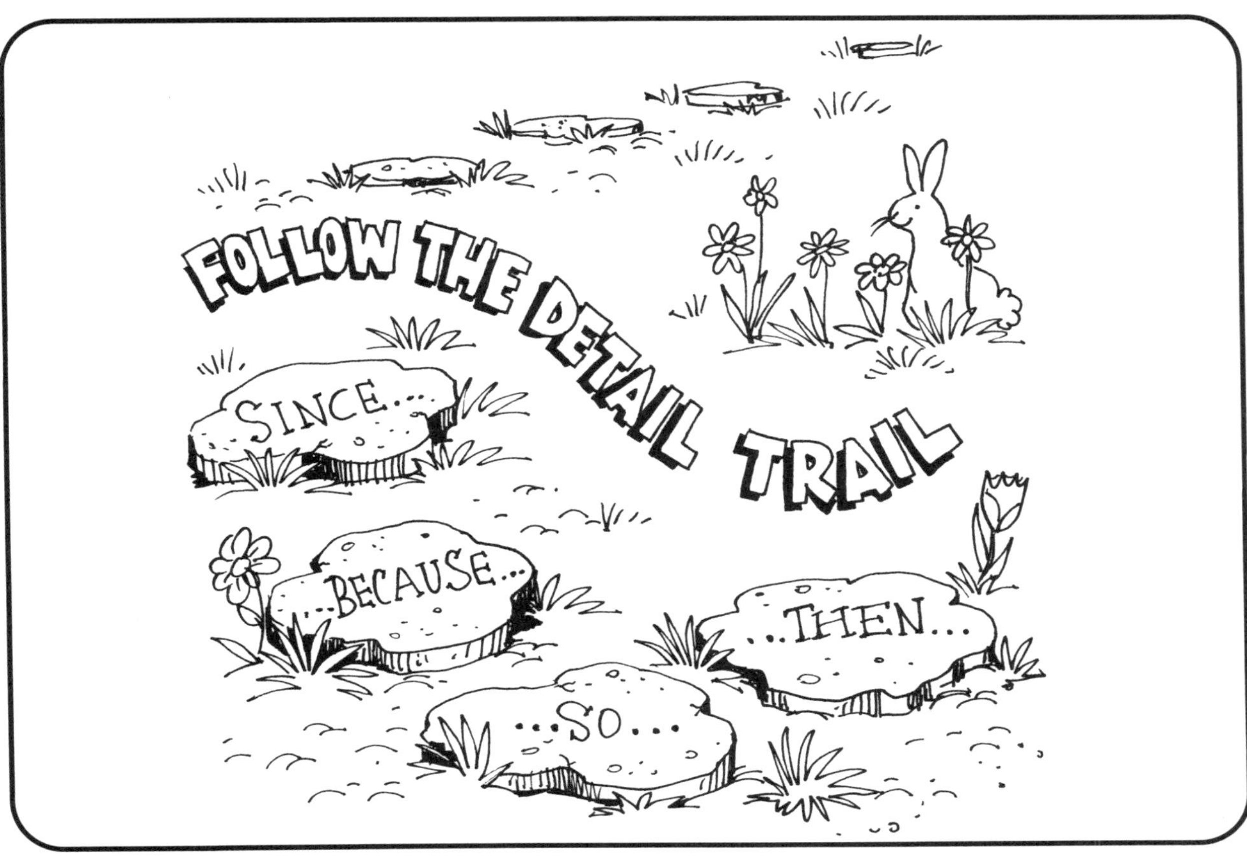

Dear Family,

1. Have your child explain the *Follow the Detail Trail* strategy and tell why it's important to recognize cause and effect.
2. Talk about three events described on the evening news. Ask your child to think of what the cause of the event was and what the effect might be.
3. Play a cause and effect game. You give the cause and have your child say the effect. Examples:
   If you eat your vegetables, ____________________.
   If you brush your teeth, ______________________.
4. If your child completes these activities, please sign below and return this form to school.

Family Member: ________________________________ Date: ______________________

STRATEGY REVIEW VACATION CALENDAR

GOAL

To maintain strategy use

BACKGROUND INFORMATION

The main focus of this lesson is to provide a way to maintain strategies in the form of home review and practice.

OBJECTIVES

1. Review and practice the language strategies.
2. Provide activities to encourage application of skills at home.

MATERIALS

1. *Strategy Guide Booklets* (One per student; assembled during the last lesson.)
2. *Vacation Calendar* (See pages 248–249; duplicate one per student.)

INTRODUCTION

Tie-in to Prior Learning

Refer to the students' *Strategy Guide Booklets* as a collection of their work throughout this school year.

Focus/Relevancy

1. Ask students to recall and tell every strategy and activity included in the *Strategy Guide Booklet.* Show the actual guide and state that it would probably be easier to use it as a reference for the year's worth of work. Hand out the students' *Strategy Guide Booklets* and instruct students to take them home.

2. Discuss the use of this strategy guide as a way to review the student's work. Having this guide will aid them in their job of being successful thinkers and communicators at school, at home, and in the community.

LESSON ACTIVITIES

1. Before duplicating the calendars, add the years, months, and days to them. Hand out the calendar pages and discuss them. Reinforce the importance of sharing this information at home, and the ease and fun of doing these assignments. Students can really impress their friends and family with what they have learned!

2. Stress that each activity takes only minutes to complete. Suggest hanging the calendars in a visible place (e.g., the refrigerator) so that students and family members will not forget to do the activities. Tell students to initial each activity when it's done. A reward for completed and initialed calendars returned after the vacation from school might encourage students to complete the activities.

CLOSURE

Summarize the lesson, review its relevance to students, and tie it to future learning. Emphasize that by practicing the activities on the calendar the students will be "ahead of the game" when they return. Say to students,

> *I hope that each of you will really be ahead of the game when we return to school after the long holiday!*

Name	MONTH	Year

Sunday	Monday	Tuesday	Wednesday	Thursday	Friday	Saturday
Turn a cartwheel! Vacation is finally here!	Tell the ***Give Me Five*** strategy.	What does it mean to compare? What does it mean to contrast?	Go to the library and check out a good book. (Tell about your favorite character!)	Tell the important story ingredients from your book!	To solve an analogy, we need to discover the __________ .	Tell at least five different verbs that describe what you do when you swim.
Go fly a kite! What must you do to fly a kite? Tell the steps.	When you don't understand something, you need to ask for __. (a long word)	If Mom says you need to "vacuum the grass," what would you do? Does it make sense?	If you wrote a story, what would be the problem in the story?	Tell the setting of your story.	How do you read the "dots" in an analogy? __ : __ :: __ : __	Eat some ice cream! Use all your senses to describe it!
Draw a picture of a cause and an effect.	Compare and contrast a watermelon and a cantaloupe.	Why would you "lasso" these words into a category? Cucumber, grass, lime, 4-leaf clover	**Keep Reading!** How would you solve the problem in the story you are reading?	Tell the story ingredients of a favorite movie.	Discover the pattern: handle : cup pedal : bike buckle : belt	Give the directions for a game to a friend and then play it together.
Make up a play about a cause and an effect.	How are Rollerblades and a bicycle alike? How are they different?	What are your five senses? Share the strategy for remembering with a friend.	Check out an adaptation of a familiar story like *The True Story of the Three Little Pigs.*	What is the problem (in the book checked out yesterday) and how do the characters solve it?	Discover the pattern: cow : pasture car : garage book : shelf	Vacation's heating up! Name three ways to keep cool in the summer.
Describe the shapes that you can see in the clouds.	Hide a toy in your bedroom. Give your friend directions for finding it.	Tell as many meanings as you can think of for the word show.				

Directions:
Initial each activity when you've done it. Save this calendar and bring it back to school after vacation.

Name | MONTH | Year

Sunday	Monday	Tuesday	Wednesday	Thursday	Friday	Saturday
What is a synonym? Tell synonyms for: hot, fast, ill, laugh, cry.	Give two meanings for the word *fly*. Can you think of any more?	Check out a book. Describe the main idea of your story.	Go for a walk in the park. Find different categories with at least three members.	Use your senses to describe fireworks on Independence Day.	Tell four words that describe how the water feels when you play in the sprinkler!	Tell a noun, a verb, and an adjective that has to do with summer.
Tell two synonyms for cold. Use them in sentences. Does the meaning stay the same?	Check out a new book. When and where does the story take place? Who are the characters?	Complete these opposites: Not morning, but___ . Not work, but ___ . Not easy, but ___.	Hit the bull's-eye by giving directions for making a peanut butter sandwich.	Ride a bike. Name six parts of a bike. (You've just made a category.)	Eat some pizza. Tell or write a descriptive sentence about it.	Watch a movie. Tell what it is mainly about. (Main character and problem)
Weigh the Meaning of these two sentences: • The water was freezing. • The water was icy.	Define the word *vacation*.	Have you read any books with a surprising outcome? Explain the outcome.	Compare and contrast vacation and school.	Name the category: 1. soda 2. pizza 3. movie (They are part of the ___ group.)	What does this expression mean? Take a "dip" in the pool.	Cause and effect: The river water was brown and smelly. What could cause this?
What might be the effects of staying out in the sun too long without sunscreen?	Use the computer in the library to find a book on mammals, reptiles, sports, or your choice.	Give two distinctive features of your favorite animal. What subcategory is your animal in?	Give antonyms for the words: 1. wide 2. quick 3. wonderful 4. found	Play with a friend. School starts soon!	Have fun! Read a good book or watch a good movie. Tell a friend about it.	Write at least two sentences showing different meanings for the words: *duck, block*.
Keep reading! Check out a book about a place you would like to visit. Tell why.	Name 10 different categories you might find in a grocery store.	Hit the bull's-eye by giving precise directions to get from your house to school.				

Directions:
Initial each activity when you've done it. Save this calendar and bring it back to school after vacation.

BIBLIOGRAPHY

A River Ran Wild (1992) by Lynne Cherry
San Diego, CA: Harcourt Brace
ISBN 0-15-200542-0

Aunt Isabel Tells a Good One (1992) by Kate Duke
New York: Penguin
ISBN 0-14-050534-2

Barn Dance! (1986) by Bill Martin Jr. and John Archambault
New York: Holt
ISBN 3-0126-00565-7975

Eye Spy: A Mysterious Alphabet (1991) by Linda Bourke
San Francisco: Chronicle Books
ISBN 0-87701-805-7

The Great Kapok Tree (1990) by Lynne Cherry
Orlando, FL: Harcourt Brace Jovanovich
ISBN O-15-200520-X

Little Sister for Sale (1992) by Morse Hamilton and Gioia Fiammenghi
New York: Cobblehill Books
ISBN 0-525-65078-4

No Moon, No Milk! (1993) by Chris Babcock
New York: Crown
ISBN# 0-517-58779-3

Possum Come a-Knockin' (1990) by Nancy Van Laan
New York: Knopf
ISBN 0-679-83468-0

Roxaboxen (1991) by Alice McLerran
New York: Scholastic
ISBN O-590-45589-3

This Is My House (1992) by Arthur Dorros
New York: Scholastic
ISBN 0-590-45302-5

REFERENCES

Asch, S., and Nerlove, H. (1960). The development of double function terms in children. In B. Kaplan and S. Wapner (Eds.), *Perspectives in psychology* (pp. 47–60). New York: International Universities Press.

Bloom, B.S. (1956). *Taxonomy of educational objectives.* New York, NY: Longman.

Caine, R., and Caine, G. (1991). *Making connections teaching and the human brain.* Menlo Park, CA: Innovative Learning Publications.

Genishi, C. (1988). *Young children's oral language development.* ERIC Clearinghouse on Elementary and Early Childhood Education, Urbana, IL. (ERIC Document Reproduction Service No. ED 301 361)

Gorman-Gard, K.A. (1992). *Figurative language: A comprehensive program.* Eau Claire, WI: Thinking Publications.

Grace, C. (1992). *The portfolio and its use: Developmentally appropriate assessment of young children.* ERIC Clearinghouse on Elementary and Early Childhood Education, Urbana, IL. (ERIC Document Reproduction Service No. ED 351 150)

Herman, J.L., Aschbacher, P.R., and Winters, L. (1992). *A practical guide to alternative assessment.* Alexandria, VA: Association for Supervision and Curriculum Development.

Hunter, M. (1982). *Mastery teaching.* El Segundo, CA: TIP Publications.

Jalongo, M. (1991). *Strategies for developing children's listening skills* (Fastback No. 314). (Available from the Phi Delta Kappa Educational Foundation, P.O. Box 789, Bloomington, IN 47402)

Johnson, D., Johnson, R., and Johnson Holubec, E. (1990). *Circles of learning* (3rd ed.), Edina, MN: Interaction Book Company.

Kavalic, S., and Olsen, K. (1993). ITI: *The model-integrated thematic instruction.* Village of Oak Creek, AZ: Kavalic.

Martin, B. Jr., and Archambault, J. (1986). *Barn dance!* New York: Henry Holt.

McInroy, J. (1996, February). *I told him 100 times!* Presentation at the Region X Educational Service Center, Richardson, TX.

McLerran, A. (1991). *Roxaboxen*. New York: Scholastic.

Naremore, R. (1995). *Language intervention with school-aged children: Conversation, narrative, and text.* San Diego, CA: Singular.

Oxford, R. (1994). *Language learning strategies: An update.* ERIC Digest. ERIC Clearinghouse on Languages and Linguistics, Washington, DC. (ERIC Document Reproduction Service No. ED 376 707)

Rief, S.F. (1993). *How to reach and teach ADD/ADHD children.* West Nyack, NY: The Center for Applied Research in Education.

Roeber, E. (1980). *Development and validation of objective referenced test instrument for critical listening: Grades 4, 7, and 10* (Technical report). Michigan Department of Education, Lansing, MI.

Wagner, B. (1989). *Whole language: Integrating the language arts—and much more.* ERIC Digest. ERIC Clearinghouse on Reading and Communication Skills, Bloomington, IN. (ERIC Document Reproduction Service No. ED 313 675)

Wiig, E., and Semel, E. (1980). *Language assessment and intervention for the learning disabled.* Columbus, OH: Merrill.